THE TRUE COST OF HEALTHCARE TODAY

A view from behind the curtain in a Massachusetts hospital

A Bezalel

Revised January 2019

TABLE OF CONTENTS

Patient: *Healthcare*

Illness*: Greed*

Diagnosis: *Hypertrophic ego*

Cure*: Non-Ado*

Therapy: *Vocation*

PRE-RAMBLE

Many presume stupid those with no interest in pettiness

I'll go right to the conclusion to save the less inclined some reading time: the true cost of health care today is our own lives collectively and individually. Keeping yourself healthy and staying away from the doctor is your best investment for a long, happy, healthy future. Please note: there is a big difference between health and wealth. Many are confused.

"He who increases his wealth by interest and overcharge gathers it for him who is kind to the poor." Proverbs 28:8

"In the beginning...God said, 'Let there be light,' and there was light." (New American Bible 1997-1998 Edition, page 8)

Now, one with a strong faith in God would not doubt the above to be truths, but, there are, no doubt, others who do. Notwithstanding, from the moment we, as humans, leave the womb, pass through the birth canal, and enter the world outside the womb, we thus come into the light.

Certainly we have no idea as to such profound physical changes as they relate to us at that major life changing moment in our own time, but, we are cast into the light—into the world, like it or not. Most of us, eventually, come to see the light, maybe not in any proverbial sense but certainly in the physical sense:

how it reflects off of objects and back onto and into ourselves.

So, from the very moment of our birth, light shines upon us. We must accept and move on into this world as we come to see it. We all come to see and interpret this life's light in many vast and varied ways. There are some things in this life we all must come to experience, such as: from the moment of inception, life is regulated by having to deal with "shit"—or "crap"—if you prefer; some may be too squeamish for the slang. Nevertheless, call it what you will, it still must be dealt with, and it all stinks. Whether we like it or not, we all must deal with the "crap" this life produces, in all its vast and varied ways. And we must deal with illnesses, sufferings, and death.

To put it another way: life is one big lesson in letting go. From beginning to the very last we must let go. It does not matter whether we learned our lessons well or not. In the end we all "pass."

To see "the light" metaphorically is another story altogether. Here I intend to shed some light on the unhealthy state of America's corporal health with which we live today: the corporate institution of "healthcare" and the hidden (or somewhat hidden) "anti-social" "crap" (in more forms than one) that go along with it.

Please note: these here before you are solely my views, thoughts, feelings, interpretations, and ideas on events I have experienced through the years. Much information is firsthand accounts and/or generalizations and information gathered through the years via many sources: written, verbal, and otherwise. Please excuse any inaccuracies, for all are just my interpretation of real-time events and events of times gone by.

Life is full of ambiguities and so to herein.

HEALTHCARE

Health care in and of itself, in the U.S., is sick and dying. The cost of health care in this country has become mindboggling, to say the least, without much, if any, improvement in overall individual and communal health. We, as a society, have gone beyond the point of either being able to afford the new technology in health care, or we, collectively, through thought and action, do not care to spend the money. As the economy limps along at the beginning of this new millennium, the populace looks to the politicians to cure its ills. All the while a large part of corporate America adds to these ills: there is money to be made in illness. Congress's law designed to give every citizen access to health care is, they all seem to agree, failing. Congress and the Administration bicker relentlessly in public view as to what is good for the country as a whole and can find little common ground but for agreeing that "one-size" does not fit all. Doctors are failing their patients when they put mammon first. Do doctors do this? Yes. I call it "doctor-centered" health care. When the doctor orders tests to protect his or herself from a lawsuit, it is doctor-centered care. The doctor is thinking about his/herself and how the orders and decisions made will affect his or her own personal reputation and financial health in the present and future. This is not the patient-centered care that we are led to believe it is. I will get further into this topic later on.

The institution of hospital is no different. The administrators practice what I like to call "bottom-line-centered" care, where it is all about making a profit. And yet we are duped into believing that some of these hospital healthcare institutions are "not-for-profit." It is just accounting "smoke-and-mirrors." I will touch further on this issue later also. We are led to believe they all are about patient-centered care. It is not true. This is like the inside joke of the medical professionals as to "practicing evidence-based" medicine. Whose evidence? The insurance companies' evidence are the numbers that direct medical care these days. There was this clipped newspaper cartoon taped on the back of the Respiratory Care Department's locker room door depicting a frustrated doctor telling a patient they have only been approved for the "second" best treatment by their insurance company.

I remember that attitudes within the hospital setting began to change when the institution's administration began instructing their health care workers to refer to the patient as "the customer." This very well may have begun on the premise to actually improve on patient-centered care but became a call for a "give the patient what they want" mentality so as to keep the revenue flowing in.

Now hospitals compete for customers. Competition in health care, how can that be? Does not every sick person deserve to be dignified with the best care out there? One institution advertises that they are better at offering particular services than another—how so?

This is some of the intermingling of money between the "healthcare" industry, the insurance industry and the tax dollar. Many predicted early on that once the "baby-boomers" became elderly, they would have a say as to the return of all their hard earned contributions at the polls. Money they had contributed to coffers over the years, destined for future health care needs, can sway a voter's line of thought. The bombast makes another entrance. Many foresaw the sums of money would be large. And like most other endeavors in life, be it noble or otherwise: where the money goes, goes the scoundrel. "Sociopath" is a noun often heard expressed between allied health workers within the halls of the hospitals these days.

The "healthcare" industry along with the insurance industry is full of them. The "Sociopath" persona is the free capitalistic social culture we have come to accept as "the norm," along with banking, high-tech, and any number of other high-financed institutions that like to bilk off or "skim" from the productive, or otherwise, hardworking community via low wages for the "worker" and high costs of goods and services to them.

First we need to get some perspective on, and define, "healthcare." What is healthcare and how did we get here?

BEGINNINGS

In the beginning, ancient texts tell us, there was good and evil. Fact or fable, it is pretty clear, once one matures and grows in years in this world, one would be hard pressed to deny that good and bad people have been around for a very long time. Cain letting Abel's blood seep into the soil has tainted the human race for a very long time. And yet, from that were born compassionate people: people who cared unselfishly for the less endowed, the sick, the infirm, and the dying.

Nevertheless, bullies and brutes continued to thrive through violence and intimidation. And, no doubt, when two bullies "square-off," someone is going to get hurt. If not the bullies themselves, surly someone in the vicinity! It has been said that African folk law states: "When two elephants fight, it is the grass that gets the worst of it."

Warring forces the reality of the times; struggling for territory—which really boils down to control of resources—was the goal toward survival. Just as in all nature, the struggle to survive is all wrapped up in 'feeding' territory. All life forms need a certain amount of 'space' with resources to sustain it. One cannot live off of inorganic matter for long. As technology advanced and progressed, the manipulation of these coveted resources advanced into destruction and devastation, of proportions never before imagined. One weapon advanced to breach another's defenses, as defenses advanced to ward off the breach. And yet compassion grew alongside the destruction, maybe even more so because of it—hope continued toward a better world. I would also imagine that along the way some of the "hope" became threadbare.

Tribes and clans grew into city-states as people began to congregate where the living was "good" with many natural resources to draw from and plenty to go around. The "free-market" was born. Along with the city-states came new illnesses and disease—much different from those found in the tribal clans, where many found themselves living the nomadic lifestyle, which certainly must have aided in the health and wellbeing of the community by not staying in one place for too long, the latter of which could, and did, cause much death and destruction of the natural habitat by human waste. Notwithstanding, nature provides the remedies and cures of the ills and sicknesses that go along with the wilderness life. Sometimes, that is. "Medicine-men" learned early on the benefit of passing on acquired knowledge, and the practice became a trade. The trade mutated just as the maladies mutated as larger and larger numbers of people began living in closer quarters: the city-state. This brings us into all-new states of illnesses and diseases, beyond the blunt-force trauma injuries, which afflicted mostly the young, healthy, physically fit adult male individuals who, grouped tightly together in close quarters, struggled with their own communicable diseases in warring times, on, and off, the field of battle no doubt. Along with all this, as much time passed, came caring/healing and, at times, cures; cures being developed, from trial and error, and observations, by the medicine men and women. But probably, more often than not, it was really just an endeavor to help reduce suffering. And yet the quest for a cure was ever present.

The city-state, or beginning "market" type of a social structure of trade brought networking, if you will, where people came and traded goods and ideas and services. The market. The birth of the "free market." The "bully" ruler came to appreciate the value of these "free markets" and the "medicine men"

12

and elevated these unique individuals into "the mystics." Magic came to be. How could Aaron turn a stick into a serpent or a river into blood? Maybe only violence could really explain such things, and the medicine men and magicians, with all their "home-brews" and sorcery, were called in to "play."

So the value of the medicinal and noble cause came to be associated with the relief of human suffering. Health care in ancient times would have been associated mostly with helping in reducing human suffering, either from illness or injury. To be sure, in those barbaric times, suffering must have been great.

Certainly as time went by many came to care for many.

COMMUNITY AT LARGE

On many levels the community at large needs the community to survive; and so it did, even thrived. Democracy became a natural thing where people and populations needed the caucus to continue to thrive and survive. The King now ruled by threat and force, sometimes cunning, and yet, as history continues to show, ultimately the people always rule. The caucus convened at times to the Church, as community, and the Aldermen, the wise seniors of the community, with their reverence and knowledge, gained by storytelling, and through heuristics came to be greatly valued. These wise people meeting at scheduled intervals, or when deemed necessary, even sought out at times by the community for rules the community might live by in harmony. The concerns by the altruistic of the commonweal gave rise to the Commonwealth, as we know it today. Everyone had their place, and vocation was the ultimate endeavor for all.

There have been, and are, many forms of social structures. People working together for a common cause of greater good, proving to be useful in numerous, nay, innumerable ways! Thus the human race has come to populate a whole lot of the grounded earth in a communal form in many ways.

Notwithstanding, fighting and warring over territory, and the resources that go along with it, have brought great minds together, if not always for a noble cause. Discoveries and the astounding human ability to adapt, communicate, record, implement, and thus thrive have shown the incredible staying power of life itself. Always has it amazed me just how many people can abuse him or herself, in one way, shape, or form, physically and/or mentally, over and over again, and still live for a very long time to tell about it. It may not be a very high quality of life but is still classified as among the living. Nevertheless, eventually, the "piper" must be paid. Sayings I've heard over the years: "There is a price to be paid for everything"; "nothing in this life is for free!" Wisdom is not in short supply; it just needs prodding much of the time. Yet, beware of advice; it has led many a well-intended soul down a dubious and slippery path.

There is much to be learned from the past, no doubt; being so vast and varied one could go on forever—and really, in some far-fetched probability—we shall. But this is for another chapter. Let's just say, people have been getting sick for a very long time, and, just as long, people have been caring for them, with hopes of relieving, or at least reducing, pain and suffering and restoring them back to a healthier state. The care and maintenance in keeping and/or the endeavors of restoring to a state of "good health" is the definition of "health care." Nevertheless, we, as a species, still keep nailing people to a cross: metaphorically speaking that is—sometimes maybe not!

Jumping into the modern era, as I've already spoken of, many of the resources concerned have been used to develop weapons of destruction to grab for more resources. Many certainly say, "What a waste." I can't say I disagree. This happens at many levels and is not the main issue other than to note the conglomeration of health care into "healthcare" and resources' redirection and how it affects the communal-social structure as a whole. Yet all this, nonetheless, adds to the human pain and suffering. On many levels!

Along with the advancements in technologic tools came the advancements in medical know-how and implementations to save and even prolong life.

The "Great" World Wars, as the World Wars' I and II misnomers have come to be known, gave way to rapid advancements in all sorts of technological know-how, some for good, some not so much—some may say just out right evil. Yet, here we are, able to keep people alive when, to all appearances, God seems to be calling them to move on into the next space. Notwithstanding, there is life after death, for many continue to live after loved ones have come and gone. Life is hard after death.

The cycles of life (and death) are truly mystifyingly complex to the living human mind, and soul.

CULTURAL RESOLUTION

Religion, as it came to be known, for some reason, seemed to draw the kindhearted to care for the sick, infirm, and dying; volunteers (religious or otherwise), out of the kindness of their hearts, as it is understood, took the charge. The scoundrel, as money and resources went in the direction of caring for the sick and infirm, also began to take notice and interest—in more ways than one. As time passed, to the institution—as these institutions of "healthcare" developed as they did—the scoundrel and their sycophants made their way. With money and resources allotted to the endeavor of caring for the sick, infirm, and dying individuals of the community, caring began to expand to the health of the whole community at large. So, in the beginning, a lot, if not relatively all, of people caring for the sick, indigent, infirm, and dying were good, kindly, caring people who would, out of the goodness of their hearts, as I've said, take it upon themselves, volunteering as it were, to care for those who were sick and dying and who had no one, or means to care for themselves. Some today would refer to the actions of these kind, caring people as givers; the returning of blessing attributes that God had bestowed upon them. Certainly these were God-fearing people, but, of course, there are always exceptions to the rule. Some care for the sole and/or soul sake of caring. It is just in their nature. Others not so much; call it what you will.

The Church: the Community: the People would set aside some space at their place of worship for the caring and comforting of the sick and destitute or infirm, maybe the basement or a shed or outbuilding of the church where they could have a dry place to lay down and die with a little less

17

suffering. The people of these close-knitted communities knew each other's faces; they could not just leave these less "blessed" or by nature, destitute, some at their own hands others by no fault of their own, to suffer and die without care. People had compassion. So the compassionate stepped in, and the community obliged. Of course there were times some communities would try to ship their troubles downstream, coming to be known as "the ship of fools." As the culture developed, they found another ship of the destitute, criminals, and the mentally deranged along with the diseased and terminally ill just upstream, headed their way. Something had to be done. Communities had to take care of their own at the very least. So the Church, the now religious segment of the social structure, stepped in with a viable plan for the problems that life cruelly casts upon us. "Is anyone among you sick? He should summon the presbyters of the church, and they should pray over him and anoint him with oil..." James 5:14 (NAB; Fireside Bible Publishers 1997-1998 edition).

TRADESMEN

The Church: the community pitched in and contributed at their weekly meetings and worships to fund the commonweal.

The priest would manage the funds, as they had been instructed to do from time immeasurable, but now the tradesmen would collect the tithing, for they knew the value in being true, level, plum, and honest: fair and square. Times change, and so do the social structures of culture—sometimes fast, other times very subtly; before you know it times have changed and yourself along with it, often times without the least bit of awareness until in the throes of a new age.

This, I suppose, may be around the time the scoundrel makes their entrance. The Sociopath, however, knows no bounds. It is an old adage handed down to our time: "if you want to find criminals, just follow the money."

I began to notice from a very early age that the banker was very often winning in the very popular board game Monopoly. I was often at a great disadvantage playing with my older brothers. They seemed to know things I did not. They seemed to always be volunteering to do the "chore" of banking for everyone else, and, more often than not, found themselves in the "winners circle," so to speak. Then, at some point, the other players would find them, the money handlers, appearing generous in helping out a fellow "player" with some donated cash to help someone out who just happened to find themselves in a financial kind of bind. Subtly and unspoken, nonetheless, beholden to the generosity, it was difficult to get out from under their influence once the generosity was accepted. Sometimes they would forgive the rent, but usually it was only discounted, for they had houses they needed to maintain. Beware of the private donors who want their names on the buildings and plaques displaying their great generosity for: "True giving is done anonymously." The tradesmen know this. The honest ones respect it. Others maybe not! Governments can debase giving with the lure of tax credits. But this is for another discussion.

We hear of private donors making large contributions for such noble endeavors, yet the majority of the funding comes from the community at large, for they knew, one day, God willing, they too will be old and in need of care—or worse, fall ill to a debilitating disease, many of which abound and strike many times without a moment's notice, the young.

As time went by and populations grew the need for caring for the sick and infirm grew also, so did the facilities with which to care for them. The hospital was born. We can trace the hospital, as an institution, developing along the way, back in history a very long time. There are biblical mentions of "hospital"; Damascus notes a hospital dating back to the 10th century. New London Connecticut's history tells of the whaling industry, which at its crest, gave to the institutions for health care. "Oil from whales and seals was exploited, yet essential to developing our industrial revolution in the 19th century. The wealth accumulated from whaling was invested in railroads, industrial development, the hospital and the creation of cultural institutions still in use today by the New London community," states a plaque, commemorating such developments, along the harbor's banks of this old and yet relatively recent sea-rearing town in the broad scope of history, as we as humans have noted it to be. We could be wrong in our views; nevertheless, I will continue in my assessment of the universe unfolding as it appears before me. I jump. But the flow is continuously moving in the direction planned out as the universe undoubtedly unfolds as it must. Time could be construed as the ultimate detractor of Godliness: evil? Maybe. Yet it has been said, "God has created all things, and all things God has created are good." Some may beg to differ. I will leave this judgment up to each of you, the reader, to his, or her, own conclusions, if any.

SOME HISTORY

One can only imagine (or not) what it must have been like not that long ago to fall ill. Many over the years have found themselves destitute at no fault of their own. Others have stepped in to help. All with their own thoughts and perceptions as to why and how. We will never know entirely for sure, if at all, what has motivated people in the past to their benevolent ways. Vocation, nonetheless, is the word applied. People—in a very crude observational way—are either givers or takers.

Certainly the caregivers of the past were givers; many did so voluntarily, as stated. The church would have parishioners go out into the community to help care for the sick and infirm. There were personal benefactors at times. Some even giving large sums of money. Some were known and, some may never be known. Nevertheless, usually the community would need to step in and care for the sickly and infirm, for it was not good policy to let people die and lie decomposing on the side of a road. This became a public health issue and so, of course, needed to be dealt with, in a rational, "health-bent" fashion, for all. So many people had helping hands in many communities of antiquity as far as their resources would allow. Things were a lot different not that long ago.

Once things started to change technologically in medicine, they changed fast. A lot of this fast-paced change came along on the coattails of war. Warfare always provides innovation on both the aggressors' and the defenders' sides. And so with medicine: as one new illness is defined, a new treatment is devised—usually only treating symptoms, not promoting a cure! Providing a cure would curtail business in today's world. We also see this with antibiotics. Bacteria, we have come to find, are very good at adapting and mutating themselves for survival. Bacteria also innovate to build up defenses. So the lab tries to come up with a new solution, literally, to defeat!

Before World War I medicine on the field of battle was not much more than stuffing linen into an open wound or sawing off limbs to head off infection and gangrene. With the manufacturing of mass-produced weaponry, bombs, and explosives with longer ranges and greater destructive power, the army hospital was expanded. Along with this expansion was the advent of newer medicines, besides alcohol (ethanol, or EtOH), for pain management, including the advent of administering intravenous fluids (IV) to manage the newly defined medical condition of "shock," the introduction of antibiotics, and the understanding and treating of sepsis. Big improvements in medicine came with the ravishings of war. The understanding of the human anatomy and its physiology improved. Artificial ventilation of the lungs with supplemental oxygen, for example, was an incredible advancement in techno-physiological know-how. Most of this advancement did not come along until right around the time electricity was harnessed and implemented for physical works. Much advancement in medicine came about rapidly in the 19th and 20th centuries. Becoming aware of microorganisms did much for the survival of the patients. The advancement and knowledge of the human anatomy through research, legal or not, on cadavers, brought about more surgeries, and with the advent of Morton's ether in the mid-1800s, and shortly thereafter nitrous oxide, the patient now could be more cooperative during a surgical procedure. Many new drugs and medications were introduced, and scientific curiosity led down many a dark ally. In the long run, however, all this new knowledge of the human species gave rise to more patients in need of care for longer periods of time. Caring for people after a surgery became more intensified, and the critical patients' needs for specialized attention rose exponentially. Thus the intensive care unit (ICU) came on the scene; personnel nursing these critical patients increased. Ratios began to change from a "nurse" caring for 5 or 10 or even more patients to a 1:1 or 1:2 nurse to patient(s) ratio becoming more the order of the day.

And, of course, the technological advancements that could not have come about without electricity created a need for more space. The cardiac monitoring of post-cardiac events became more in use and improved rapidly. The extraction of medical oxygen to be administered as a drug became a normal occurrence within a very short time. However, like many technological advancements through the events of history, the adverse effects became known only over time and through experimentation with willing (and sometimes not) participants. Some practitioners may have been overly zealous in their excitement of discovering a new panacea, a "cure-all," that safety may not have been first on their minds.

But, like free oxygen radicals and the havoc they can play with molecular biological forces, many new discoveries regarding molecular derangement were, and still are, not well respected or understood, and, when used irresponsibly in the medical professions, can turn deadly—as if there would be no side effects to large amounts of high fractionally inspired oxygen (FiO2). The advent of mechanical ventilation would never have come about without the development of compressing gases and moving these gases within closed circuits—first with the negative driving pressures like the Iron Lung to the positive-pressure ventilator providing support for patients with a compromised respiratory drive, for whatever reason, induced or otherwise. Now this very brief and far from complete walk through time with regard to medicine and its devices gives us some perspective as to really how new "advanced" medicine is. We are on the cusp of discovering amazing things in relation to the human body and its environment. I foresee extra corporal membrane oxygenation (ECMO) becoming so advanced that people with advanced stages of chronic obstructive pulmonary disease (COPD) will be able to function much more freely with "hand-held" pocket devices that will only need something like a tiny computer chip periodically replaced to replenish depleted catalyst molecules (which extract oxygen (O_2) from the carbon dioxide (CO_2) in the blood), bypassing the lungs altogether. The opportunities are endlessly unfathomable today. Tomorrow will seem silly what we know today as "advanced." Like the telephone today as to when it first came on the scene—when the first crank phone with its finely polished wooden box and metal-crank and a horned tube attached to talk into and another on a string to listen to, was real fine stuff back in the 1800s. Some real fine workmanship and engineering, but of course the big news was who it was connected to some distance away.

Anyway, this gives us a little bit of history and allows us to keep in perspective where we are, to some extent, and where we have been, and, with regards to some indulgence in a bit of artistic liberty, some future imaginings. For without a healthy imagination we would, with all probability, never be here.

PERSONAL BACKGROUND

Now I must give the reader a little bit of my own background to place things a tad more into perspective and cast a light on how I have come to write this narrative. In 1980 I entered a respiratory therapy certification program at a nearby community college. At that time one would study two three-month semesters in a classroom setting then a three-month semester "interning" in a local hospital setting, treating patients based on the classroom knowledge acquired just prior. I refer to this as "slave-labor," for we were required to work 40 hours per week, eight hours a day, five days a week, Monday through Friday, without pay. How does one survive such a venture? I worked evenings and weekends at odd jobs, just as most college students of the day, to supply income to eek out a marginal existence.

After my "internship" I was offered a job at this hospital where I had interned and, desperate for a living wage—not that this new job was a living wage at $2.22 per hour—it was a move up from no pay at all, and I took the job instead of continuing one more year of education (2 semesters in class and one more in-house). So began a 36-year career in the allied health "industry." I did not realize, at the time, that it was such an industry! Maybe it wasn't or maybe I was just too young and naive to know at that time.

I worked at a trauma I teaching hospital, in Massachusetts, spending many years in all the aspects of medicine a large institution has to offer in the way of advanced medicine. I moved as a respiratory practitioner from assisting at high-risk deliveries to chronic elder care and everywhere in-between, but practiced mostly in the emergency rooms, cardiac ICU, trauma ICU, pediatric ICU and pulmonary/medical ICU.

MORALE

The *Harvard Business Review* published an article some time ago about how when morale is low in the workforce of a large institution, it is usually a clear indication that there is pillaging going on from above. Morale, in the healthcare industry today, is so low one hears about it daily just roaming the halls of the healthcare institutions: hospitals—from doctors, to nurses, to allied health workers, to kitchen and housekeeping help. Everyone is disgruntled about their work conditions of short staffing and short supplies yet the Board of Directors and upper management walk away with handsome pay raises and bonuses to manage profits in these "not-for-profit" institutions. Not for profit? Really? It is easy, as I've noted, to spend other people's money; easy, for some, to put a little extra into their own pockets. For one who regularly reads the news, this is old news.

The sociopathic culture began to focus on a "money-grab," infiltrating health care creating "healthcare" and began to arrange the development of the hospital as an institution.

On other fronts: It is hard to say your last goodbyes to a loved one. Most are not prepared. I have watched many bedside vigils, with lots of tears, pain, grieving, and sadness; crying, screaming, and frantic antics from the depth of emotion rising to the surface and scaring the crap out of most of the other patients and family members as to the cruel realities of life and death in the ICU.

The purging of long-internalized guilt is a sad thing to witness—bridges burnt and then doused with tears in the hopes of salvaging the ruins. I see a lot of guilt come out through the words "I love you" in the ICU. I see many patients tortured by their "loved ones" (healthcare proxy) by not giving the "OK" to let the patient (e.g., mom or dad) go. Leaving the patient literally rotting in their bed. Rotting flesh has a very unpleasant, repulsive "sweet" smell of death. Have you ever smelled living flesh begin to rot? It is horrible, and yet in this day and age it is a smell often accompanying the ICU environs.

So we, many times, as allied health professionals, per doctor's orders, keep patients alive for longer than seems humane; fear of the unknown is a strong motivator to emotional dearth. All the while, all indications being that they, the patient, are screaming for release from the profound unmitigated pain and suffering that nothing in this life can relieve, short of death: the "sweet release." Be nice to your children while they are growing up, for the day may come when they hold the trigger to the pump that administers your pain relief. Many are sadistic right to the last.

Depending on perspective, like the doctor's unknown fear of a malpractice lawsuit, one would be wise to remember: we live in a get-rich-quick, litigant-crazed society. Some families have no scruples and have no problem throwing little junior, or grandma, for that matter, under the bus, so to speak, just for a quick buck.

There have been times where it appears family members are taking the fentanyl patches off of their loved ones in the bed and using them for their own personal 'highs' letting the 'loved' one in the bed suffer great pain unnecessarily. Hard to believe!

Another case is fraud via over-billing: when one can say, "we ran all the tests and here are the objective results. There is nothing more we can do"; it absolves the doctor and hospital of having to withstand increasing liability insurance premiums and, at the same time, increases revenue. A double positive for the medical profession! But, in the end, we all pay; one way or another we all pay. Now let's shuffle those funds around, shall we.

FUNDS

The Wall Street Journal published an article back in the 70s about the large amounts of money flowing into the Federal Medicare/Medicaid healthcare system by the then baby-boomers entering the workforce. It was stated how, when elderly, this population will, most likely, swing some weight at the polls in how the money will be spent. I don't know if this, in fact, has come to pass, but what I have observed is that the sociopath has infiltrated health care for "healthcare" is now where the money is! A Harvard educated, professional financial planner once said to me how "the money is out there, you just need to find out where it is." And I say: if you want to find out where the money is, just look for the scoundrels: the sociopaths.

As many of the "baby-boomers" were beginning to open their eyes to their very own mortality, they began to shift hard-earned money—realizing: "this isn't really the land of milk and honey"—into accounts for future health care needs that they themselves may need upon entering old age. Many felt that money that has gone into the social-governmental structures, set up to provide the funds for such health care services might not be there when the time comes to collect. They have been right. Social Security is on the brink of bankruptcy. The money 'grab' from politicians who have no shame in spending other people's money have drained the coffers and now a few are required to pay for the many; a difficult burden to be passing along to future generations. Politicians bombast their constituency for votes hiding behind pseudo-integrity. Congressmen and -women would be asked to pass laws to guarantee such care. The point being: it has been known for quite some time now that much money would flow into the coffers earmarked for health care. And "healthcare" has taken note.

Health care turned "Healthcare" seems to be moving in the direction of limiting resources so upper management's salaries can be maintained, such as: after a certain age no more computed tomography (CT) scans. I have read that some countries already have limits on these resources, claiming there is just not enough to go around. Is this the new triaging of medicine? Who gets the test or procedure and who does not? In some places healthcare systems are "life-limiting" care (testing and treatments and things of this nature) in some sort of fashion, like maximum numbers in a period of time, either to the individual patient or an institution. I've been told this is happening now in this country with dentistry and third-party payments. Lifetime spending limits, I'm lead to believe, have been implemented.

SOCIAL PATHOLOGY

"Money" can change a culture

Common business practice today is: once the sociopathic ways of an institution are found out by the people it was set up to serve, the rule is to change the name of that institution and continue the dupe under the guise of a new entity. The same old game under a new name!

Healthcare today, in the 21st century, is no longer a community service caring for the health and wellbeing of its people—the "people" of the community, which includes healthcare workers too. Healthcare has become a money-grinding machine. A "money-mill" if you will. Healthcare has become a prime economic mover within the cities of North America. Here in Massachusetts "HealthCare" is the largest employer in some broad areas of Massachusetts, according to some local Chamber of Commerce chapters, for the year 2016. Some of these institutions are "Trauma I" emergency medical institution serving Massachusetts, offering services beyond what smaller community hospitals can, or even hope to offer. These large institutions have a huge impact on area economies, providing "healthcare" to the surrounding towns and beyond. This brings a lot of insurance money and tax dollars by way of social-service systems, such as Medicare and Medicaid; here in Massachusetts the government program is called "MassHealth." The "health" institutions that do not turn sick people away certainly are commendable—I find it hard to believe that some hospitals do turn people away, but they do. There is some agreement with the State with these hospitals to take in uninsured sick people, treat them, care for them, and then track them all at the expense of the State, aka: the tax payer. These institutions, which like to hide behind the trappings of bureaucracy, channel much of the revenue back into the community through avenues such as advertisements and other such ancillary services, be it construction necessary for expansion projects or just maintenance and upkeep. It all requires wo/man-power, keeps people employed. Yet, when the "scoundrels," hiding behind institutional bureaucracy, snake their way to the top, the scale balance tilts in some unsettling ways.

Why is healthcare advertising in the first place? Are they competing for "customers?" This certainly tells us something of the culture in which we find ourselves today. The healthcare institutions are about making money. Many of the long-term "trench" workers see and know this, such as doctors, nurses, and many of the ancillary workers of the healthcare institutions. But we all have bills to pay, and most will not "bite the hand that feeds them." Revenue is the way to pay those bills.

Waste has been problematic in large institutions, and healthcare, just like any other business, is no exception. It, I believe, is always a good thing to keep waste in wraps, so to speak, but when one trims the wick too closely, the risk of snuffing-out the whole flame of an operation becomes ever present, whether one sees it or not. We see lots of ads in newspapers, billboards, banners, and civic gatherings like AARP conferences on employment and health information sessions where these "health" institutions advertise as great services and accomplishments in caring for the community. Marketing?!

The business people who run some of these large healthcare organizations are well versed in the magic of marketing. "If we tell them it is so, they will believe us." Maybe. Why compete for patients? Much money is spent on convincing the communities that these large medical institutions are providing the community with the best possible health care anywhere in the world and of just how great of an employer they are. Let me tell you: they do not and are not, on many levels. "It," today, here in the USA, is all about the money. These "healthcare" institutions are all about the money. Adam Smith tells us something about the velocity of money in a free market economy and how its value is closely tied to the health of the market. This money-market economy does not really look into how the money may be spent but for goods and services. Marketing leads us like the ring in the nose of the bull.

Historically, over and over again, we begin to see a pattern arise: with the money comes the scoundrel. Now these "money-people," people who evaluate and assess their self-worth based on the dollar, know the value of a good education and learn quickly, within the halls of academia, the great powers of "market-manipulation" via advertising, aka: marketing. Many of these large hospital institutions have been tooting their own horn for some time now, like say, as one of the top "10 healthcare providers in the country." Many employees over the years have wondered: "says who?" Most, if not all, who have been working within the hallways and trenches know the truth. These business people calling "the shots" either are really clueless as to the poor quality of health care they are providing or just do not care. Yet, they go about "lying" their way to the top of the purse strings. As noted: morale is low among the workers.

Health care, ironically, today is, on the whole, sick and dying. However, on the other side of the same coin the institution of healthcare, the hospital, is healthy, vibrant and growing very nicely for those in the top offices. These 'top-dogs' are growing fat telling people they are sick and in need of healthcare. They, management, do not care about the patient but for the dollars that can be extracted from accounts, adding to the glut of high-end salaries. It is one of today's social diseases most in need of a cure. And needed fast.

The most effective and efficient way to this end is getting the community healthy. And yet there is no money for true health care, as it is set up today, in this model. If everyone were healthy within the community, then "healthcare" would be, in many ways, out of business. These "healthcare" institutions, along with the social culture, of today are in the way of making people sick, or at the very least making them think they are sick, to insure a good "customer" base well into the future—all being funded by the "State": the taxpayer and insurers. Ultimately we, the people, the dwindling hard working healthy ones, are having to pay more and more of hard earned income to fund the accounts of those who do not.

First, one must diagnose the disease, then the cause; in this case the disease is greed. Greed! The organ infected must be identified: upper management. The concern at this point in time is how far the disease has spread to other areas of the body? Not all, as of yet, have been infected with greed. There are still many in healthcare today that truly care about the patient, but they are, to use a pun-ish phrase, a "dying breed." As we are beginning to see today, many of the people entering the healthcare professions are attracted by the "benefits" and pay offered by these professions in comparison to others, with minimal education on many levels. It is a very scary reality when dealing with people's lives: "a little bit of knowledge can be a very dangerous thing." We'll talk more on this later. Let's just say, just as with all professions and in all walks of life, there is a whole lot of incompetence out there. The scary thing is: very many do not see it until it is too late, and even then, many times, refuse to recognize it, or just don't care. People are very adept at placing the blame somewhere far from "thy-self." This is surly self-preservation, for the ego plays a huge role in identity and many, if faced with "their" true reality, would suffer greatly in seeing their very own true self exposed. Notwithstanding, there is still hope.

What type of cultural social structure goes about selling products to its citizens that makes them sick and chronically ill and then goes about selling products to treat the symptoms? History is now revealing a capitalistic social structure with a "free-market" mentality is just the type.

Another irony of today's culture is that the manufacturers of the United States today produce goods—no matter where produced—and services that have a very limited life span. They call this "quality control": duping the unawares that they are selling quality when in fact they are limiting quality to a limited life span so as to be able to sell more of the same product to the same customer at a future date, say five or 10 years; "durable goods" in business jargon. I will not go deep into the numbers of the national gross domestic product (GDP), for many have delved into that quagmire, and the information is easily ascertained for the laymen's review. Let me just state here: we base the whole health of our society on the crap that we produce. It is of no wonder that this society is so unhealthy. As I've often heard myself exclaim, "we are what we consume!" Lifestyle is everything.

In recent years some have tried to bring this aberration into the light and address it, but most do not want to see it. Why? Because most people are duped into thinking they cannot live without this crap that is being produced and pushed down the throat, so to speak. All in the name of progress. Marketing!

Now don't get me wrong, some of the products produced in this country are very useful and have helped improve, on a highly valued level, I dare say, the quality of our lives—like, for instance, indoor plumbing, hot running water and central heating, to name a few. The shower has been a major step forward in the health and wellbeing of the community at large. The washing machine has liberated people from many hours of hard, time consuming, work and toil to be spent elsewhere. But much of the stuff produced is life-limited, and limiting, crap. The irony is that "capitalists" have us paying to bring this crap into our houses, and then, when the product has met the limited life designed within it, we must pay to have it removed from our homes. Who is it that runs and operates these home rubbish removal companies? Who? Who controls the garbage, trash, and landfills and incinerators? I'll let you answer these questions for yourselves. Healthcare has come to the same. We consume the product of that which we produce, it makes us sick, we enter healthcare, and they run many tests and find other issues, which "must be treated and followed up on," the doctor tells us. "Take these pills and see me in two weeks." Feeding on fear, now you're in the system. You are not getting out alive. But unlike the quality control of the industrial inanimate "widget"—where life is limited—life must now be preserved in order to extrapolate all that cash sitting in those health insurers and tax payers coffers: a steady stream of revenue from the living patient, as long as they stay "sick and dying" and do not die too soon. At least not until the money has all been spent.

TRUTH

Pilate asks: "What is the truth?" The truth? We find the truth within ourselves, and more often than not we do not like what we find, if we even so dare as to look. Many, I imagine, care not to look at all. Most people cannot stand to look in the mirror for fear of seeing their true selves. I repeat to make the point. Metaphorically speaking that is. So to the useless crap we direct our attentions to distract us from our pathetic petty lives, and ourselves, and pretend we are happy. Please rest assured, I know of which I speak: I project. Am I not a product of this "culture" in which I live? Money has shaped my life, too, for, without it, in this culture, one cannot live. Is this why we chase after so many distractions? The fancy automobile (we cannot even afford to buy; we lease), the lavish vacation (borrowing to enjoy today what we will try to pay for tomorrow), the new computer or Smartphone! The list goes on. And on and on! The carrot swinging in front of our faces giving us the illusion of gain when in reality it is the debt-laden credit cards that keep us running in the direction, which "THEY" tell us, is "right." It seems always just out of reach to pay off the principal, so we are "allowed" to pay interest only. Sweet! Sweet for whom; Do the "moneyed class" take from the ones who are truly concerned about helping the ones in need? Indeed, from the ones *in* need? This is a "free-market capitalist" society in which we find ourselves, and we must keep this in mind as we trudge through the muck. Teddy Roosevelt might say, "Get a big rake."

And the "capitalists" love it: "give us your hard-earned money; go into debt; we'll lend you the cash." All the better, for, then, they own you, for all of your productive years—30-year mortgages are no arbitrary thing. And for what, producing what? I'm not saying we should not enjoy nice things in life, but to go into debt for such things might not be such a good idea. Some might even equate this to selling one's soul, and I might tend to agree; this is not true happiness, and yet it is by design.

Wealth and health are two totally different things. Some might argue that debt is a good financial tool used to advance one's financial stability: leverage. And, to an extent, I agree! Leverage is not a bad thing. With inflation factored into the system's economy, it only stands to reason that on a 30-year note we are paying back, on the tail end of the loan, (ideally) with easier, cheaper (devalued) money. That is: inflation has given us a little hedge, a perceived higher hourly rate of monetary compensation for our "manual" labors. So, to use a phrase: "we get more bang for our buck." That is if prices remain the same. However reality dictates that they do not. Taxes continue to rise. After a time though, it takes less of our disposable income to pay the mortgage. Of course one would have to factor in the interest paid over the years on that note and taxes, insurances, and other costs. But, in setting the stage, I digress.

In healthcare, however, it is a different story. Health care, as I have said, is sick and dying. The illness: greed. And greed likes it just as that: sick and dying, not dead, but sick and dying—preferably a long and drawn out death, if one has the money, of course. The institution of the hospital is a place for caring for patients, and the "patient," as revenue, has given the noun "customer" a whole new meaning. There is no money in death for the healthcare industry, only for the undertaker. The hospital is working toward the dream of Samuel Clemens, where even the undertaker is saddened upon the death of a person who dies penniless. In some realms, specifically the healthcare industry, business is defining "health care" via marketing, not through "caring."

The sad part is this is not by nature, *per se,* but by design—by design to make money. Do not be duped by the sales pitch of "not-for-profit" nomenclature these institutions like to throw at you. The "new-wave" educated are the sociopaths who are "money-mongering marketers" and have been well educated in the art of deception. Or more specifically: the art of marketing as noted above. These hospital administrators are sociopaths who have come to view the hospital as a vehicle to handsome incomes for themselves. The individualistic culture of the modern day "first-world!" They hide behind the guise of caring but in reality are sneering. Sociopathic capitalism. Free-market capitalism without moral fiber is the root of the problem. Commonweal has been perverted into "Common-hell!" Is this all we have to hope for in a free democratic society, of which we're taught, from an early age, to love and aspire to fame and fortune? At any cost! Is this what "community" is all about? I think not. Certainly this "dog-eat-dog" mentality comes with a price. No matter what ideology you want to play, be it socialism, communism, or some other ingenious 'dupe' sociologic-ideology; when it really comes down one finds lack of morals and ethics; undying quests for more within a framework of unethical dimensions. A perverted schema if you will. The vast majority of the population is now, and into the foreseeable future (if there even is such a thing), destined to be left out in the cold. It is easy to see how these top administrators justify their grab for capital: "we worked hard, got a good education, worked our way up through the ranks, and justly deserve to be well compensated for our efforts," they tell us. I like to call it the "Don't hate me 'cause I'm beautiful" mentality. This advanced society of "better living" is killing us. This is not some accident, but by design.

41

With all the "good" living we enjoy; it is making us sick. It is difficult not to overindulge in the land of plenty. And when sick, where do people go? The hospital emergency room very often! That's where. This is where the irony of society sucks the last few drops of life-giving blood right out of those who attend. Please do not confuse this as being akin to the noble cause of giving blood voluntarily to help save a life. Now don't get me wrong—medicine has made great advancements and helped to improve the quality of many people's lives. When handled responsibly, by which I mean with a moral and ethical structure sincerely promoting a better quality of life for all, a real positive outcome can and has ensued. Yet, and I repeat for effect, it seems that technology in medicine has advanced past our ability, and/or willingness, to pay. The Scoundrels demand their cut first and foremost.

Let's take a look at the opium epidemic, for example. We all are seeing firsthand, and reading about, almost daily, in the local and national news: ordinary hard working people turning to heroin because now it is easier and cheaper to "come by." After becoming addicted to doctor-prescribed pain killers, following some unforeseen mishap, like say, the young man from Maine who suffers a knee injury playing hockey, turns to the healthcare "industry," as most do, for treatment and rehabilitation, hoping to play hockey once again someday. And, probably just as innocently, the doctor, in the routine treatment, prescribes pain management via chemicals: pain medication. One needs to understand there are many components and many vast and varied reactions by each individual to chemicals in vivo in the making up of organic compounds we call vitality. Not everyone reacts the same way, and it is difficult to know "what is what" when it becomes a subjective disposition. Like the alcoholic—who, when a young person, going out with their friends for a good time, has that first beer—never would have thought they would find themselves, years later, face down in the gutter: a victim to alcoholism. Nevertheless, pain management is about managing pain. Pain, as it is, within the human experience, consumes a lot of energy: a lot of oxygen—oxygen that would otherwise be used in the metabolic healing process of the organic unit as a whole. It is wise to keep the pain at bay, but, to be clear, pain is nature's way of saying, "hold on a minute, you need to lay off of that injury for a while and let it heal." When we use chemicals to take the pain away, we are more prone to reinjure and create a more difficult injury to treat and cure, and possibly cause more and some real lasting irrevocable damage, if it hasn't been done already. It is pretty clear how most of these victims (and they are victims) are victims of greed. Victims of the money-grubbers, whose material needs far exceed, in their reality, the needs of the sick and suffering. More, more, and still more lose their lives while still among the living.

After all, it is the "American" way to forge ahead of the majority to boasting rights of wealth. That is: *wealth* not *health*. This is a very important point; the two should not be confused and grouped together, as today they most often are. There is a BIG difference between health and wealth. One cannot buy one with the other. Now don't get me wrong; I do believe you can have one with the other, but time tells me wealth is not a prerequisite to health *per se*. The paradox is, however, that you can have wealth through health. In my view: HEALTH is WEALTH, of the best kind, for without health, just like hope, you have nothing, or very little at most. Now I must be clear at this point: wealth is not about money, just as education is not about money specifically. Education is about quality of life. Many will disagree with me on this point due to the fact that, in this US of A, we are fed the illusion that higher education brings wealth.

43

But again, this is delusional, for wealth does not necessarily bring good health and happiness. But it can, if gone about in the right way: with a "healthy" attitude.

I'll give you a simple example: I was working late one night in the cardiac ICU, and a patient had undergone a routine open heart surgical procedure (yes they are pretty much routine these days), but something in the operating room (OR) must have gone wrong or fate had a contrary design. The patient, a successful cardiac surgeon himself, was not waking up post-op. [Cardiac patients go directly from the OR to the cardiac ICU, bypassing the recovery room (RR) in this institution] As time went on, it became clear that something was amiss with this patient. I do not remember the specifics of the case; it may have been an anoxic event (lack of oxygen to the brain for a period of time causing death of brain tissue)—not a good thing, ever.

[Things that happen in the OR stay in the OR and are seldom, if ever, revealed: bad for statistics, and bad statistics are bad for reimbursements and reputation and endowments. NO ONE EVER DIES IN THE OR!

I have witnessed cardio-pulmonary resuscitation (CPR) performed from the OR through the halls—someone actually kneeling up on the bed performing cardiac chest compressions on the patient as the bed is being wheeled down the hall, hastily and frantically, into the elevator, up to the ICU, where then the patient is pronounced dead. Death in the ICU; NEVER the OR!]

This cardiac surgeon's prognosis now is grim to hopeless, and the family, understandably so, is distraught. Frantic, really! They could not understand how a successful cardiac surgeon—my take on it—no matter being their dad, who has had a stellar career, extending the years of countless people's lives, is destined to die of a cardiac surgery himself. Oh the pathetic ironies of life. I think he was probably in his fifties. No one is exempt. This is something many people find hard to accept. This is why the Bible tells us to always keep our house in order; you never know when your time will be up. Tell your loved ones you love them while on your way out the door. It may come to pass you'll not have the chance again.

The daughters of this particular case were so upset and distraught over their father's totally unexpected turn of events, they went frantically running and screaming up and down the hallways of the cardiac ICU to the point where one of them passed out from hysteria, I suppose, and hit the floor hard. Now, not only do we have a difficult cardiac case on our hands but a trauma in the hallway to boot.

It seems to me everyone who reads enough history, and ancient texts, eventually comes to realize: folly leads to madness, and madness is folly. When one starts to realize just how short this time we, as humans, have to spend, in this form we call life, one begins to realize the actual imaginary roles we lead, deluding ourselves of our own self-professed import. We, I like to think, most of us anyway, come to realize, eventually, that pride is humility turned upside down. Pride, the Bible, in various places and ways, teaches of its folly. We, in this occidental society, pride ourselves in our accomplishments. The astronomer, on the other hand, tells us we fool ourselves into thinking we can continue on this path of existence. We cannot! Nowhere is it said the world will last forever, and we are fools of folly to think it will. On the other hand we like to think there is life after death. I could easily fall into the trap of immortality or, at the very least, the view of youthful invincibility; many believe: "youth is wasted on the young." Ignorance is not conclusive. One might come to the conclusion that we live in a world of wondrous perpetuity. The small-minded would like to live forever; the broad-minded say, "enough is enough; let me go."

Within the realm of medicine today doctors, who, I'm pretty sure have deluded themselves too, on a very broad scale, believe what it is they often tell their patients—we can save your life—leading one to think, with the doctor's expertise, we as humans have the potential to live forever. It really should not take a book to inform you: we cannot. The doctor may, however, argue the point. Doctors are not trained in the art of dying; they are trained in the art of healing (or are supposed to be, anyway). Medicine is about improving and lengthening quality of life and reducing, to the best degree possible, sufferings. Sometimes, however, life itself says: "enough is enough." So with this we need a definition of "medicine."

MEDICINE

What is it? Medicine today seems to have multiple definitions and has become today in this United States a money-making scheme. In a free society it seems to be set that the "privileged" class outweighs the less fortunate in many ways, but in the way of medicine it has come to the point where if the privileged (the ones who have come to control the resources) tell us something is true, we believe it. If the doctor says, "we can save your life," most people will believe it or, at the very least, want to believe it. Sometimes it is reality...but only in the sense as prolonging life, for better or worse. So really it comes down to quality of life. This is a very subjective avenue and not an easy one to navigate. Family and friends have their own convoluted interpretations of quality-of-life and medicine. Culture certainly plays a large role. Oftentimes, even though many have tried to address these issues currently as well as in the past, not many think to ask the one who is facing the reality of death what their definition of "quality-of-life" is. Most people, practically speaking, are not prepared for death. So medicine they seek. The fear of the unknown keeps us asking the doctor to keep us alive. And the doctor, most of them today anyway, not all, but a good number, dupe us into inflating the doctor's purse.

Today, with large corporations and institutions, we find it is the bottom line that is the focus of close care, not the patient. Those who kick and scratch their way to the top of the corporate ladder have come to dupe even the doctor of medicine to be used as a tool for the madness to "riches." This is the free society we live in. This is medicine today in America. Clearly, as a society, we

47

are all in this together so, let's get together and help each other out to improve the quality of life for the many, not just the few.

As we venture back in time, we do not, in the big scheme of things, have to go very far to find the ship of fools as I've alluded to earlier. As we sail along with the fools we find nowhere to go: up and down the rivers, out along the shores, and into the vast expanses of the open ocean. Time goes by, and these ships, exhausting their destinations, turned madhouse for medicine to advance. The community took charge and medicine came to be. Responsible for all its citizens the community took them in, cared for them, and gave them something to do, maybe. The community—in old times the Church or congregation, which entailed the whole of the populous—felt it prudent to set aside some of the tithing to care for these "lost souls," to feed them, clothe them, and keep them from causing trouble. Many seemed to think, at the time, these poor unfortunate souls had lost their minds. Some may have, at the time, thought differently. Conveniently, as the leper population diminished throughout Europe anyway, the leprosarium, the Lazar House— as Foucault likes to call them—turned into the madhouse, to fill a void nonetheless, and then on to become the clinics of medicine. The Church continued and the madness too. Folly brought many to the point of madness in their pursuits to a medicinal cure. So we come to the modern day institution of the hospital where medicine rules for which, for the sake of mammon, the administrators have sold their own souls with the illusion of the greater good. Have they gone mad? In reality, however, these "well-educated" were not taught the realities of a profound life and its transformation in ending. Becoming the madmen themselves, without knowing; having sold themselves short, if you will, in their scheming to extrapolate cash from the community at large for their own personal gain. This is a free society devoid of God, as the ancients knew of and sociology teaches today. I don't know why these well-educated administrators of today have missed this boat and are destined to ride the ship-of-fools. When their time comes, there will be no beds upon which to rest their weary heads for *"He who increases his wealth by interest and overcharge gathers it for him who is kind to the poor." Proverbs 28:8*

INSTITUTIONALIZED

As I've explained above, in the beginnings, it was, in health care, the "caring" and kind people who took in and helped those sick and dying, who, by no fault of their own, found themselves, at times, not having means of support. Some do fall to the waysides of society at no fault of their own, no doubt, and can use a helping hand. Others make poor life choices and fall into unhealthy lifestyles. Knowingly or not doesn't all that much matter, for the most part, once illness sets in.

Now it is the institutions in these United States that does the 'caring.' We are born in institutions, we are raised and educated in institutions, many work in institutions and, more often than not, most of us die in institutions. Medical institutions are where we now, in most cases, begin our lives and end our lives. In many cases it has become criminal if a loved one falls ill and one does not seek the medical professions' advice and follow recommendations to treat. It does not matter what the parent thinks in many instances. "You do not go against the doctor, for the doctor knows all" is the mentality of today's society in the West. This is "herd" mentality I say and not necessarily a healthy one for some like to take advantage of the unawares.

Unfortunately the doctors of today are, more often than not, the minions of Corporate America. Just as unsettling for many is the seeming appearance of elected officials sway alongside big business. Government was put in place in this country to protect the "little ones"— those less naturally endowed to protect themselves from the unscrupulous scoundrel—but now complaints of a corrupted electorate catering to the capitalists corporate free-world of grabbing resources abound. And to what end? All "healthcare" institutions today, more often than not, are in a sad state of affairs. To die in a cold and sterile environment surrounded by strangers seems, to me, unsettling and inhumane. To be with someone strange to you, left to die alone is a heart-wrenching experience. "Left alone" to me means without loved ones, family and friends, around. Maybe some might take comfort in caring for the sick and dying, but today, in the institutions, it is not only the bed linens and walls that are sterile; it is, very often, the staff, too, that have become sterile: "Just another day at the office," or, if you will, "in the lab," for working in an ICU is really working in a "live" laboratory at best. All of the treatments are very often really just experiments to add to the knowledge of medicine. Doctors will try different treatments and therapies based on what may have worked toward a cure in the past for patients or even themselves, but, in the real world, everything is very often subjective. What works on one is not guaranteed to work on another. So we therefore refer to the physician as "practicing" medicine. The hospital is the playing field, because, frankly, with all due respect and awe for the advancements medicine has made, doctors do not know what they are doing half the time. And that is being generous! Now of course not all doctors are phonies, but many just seem to be faking it. One would be wise to remember that arrogance is just a mask ignorance hides behind when the ego gets in the way. Many working in the allied health fields have heard coming out of their own mouths: "What do they teach these doctors in medical school? 'Cause it sure as hell doesn't seem like they are teaching them medicine!" So "practice" it is!

Bullies and cheats are now running these medical institutions for the greater good of themselves. These "bullies," hiding behind

51

bureaucracy nowadays, cause many of our illnesses; the medical profession even has a fancy name for these illnesses caused by their very own establishments: iatrogenesis.

Infections, induced addictions, unnecessary procedures leading to other unnecessary procedures, collateral illnesses are all a steady stream of revenue for the institutions; these are just some among many avenues of which I write.

Here is an example of the "death institutions" we have for ourselves today. Not many are exempt from residency in these institutions. When my elderly grandmother was placed into an assisted-living facility—much to her chagrin, and mine—I went to visit her and see how she was doing. She was making do but clearly she did not really want to be living among strangers at this stage in her advanced-age in life. She wanted to be surrounded by family, as most of us do, young and old alike. I walked with her around the facility. It was very nice. We went to sit in the lobby for a while and look out the window at the beautiful flowers growing all around outside. It is nice to be surrounded by vibrant living beings. As we are sitting talking I notice a lot of the residents are shuffling into the lobby area and just kind of mulling around. I asked my "Grams" what the entire crowd was about, for, by this time there was quite a number of residents congregating around the area where there were massive double doors closed and locked. "What are they doing?" I asked.

"Oh they are waiting for the cafeteria to open for dinner!"

We get up from our nice window seat and begin to move in the direction of the crowd when the doors swing open, and the crowd of elderly people consolidate and squeeze through the not-so-small doorway yet because of the size of the crowd it became snarled. As we are now shuffling along ourselves an older lady, a resident of the institution heading to eat, turns to me and says: "See this is what they do to you when you get old. You wait; they will do it to you, too! They stick you in here and forget all about you. You will see."

Not long after this visit my family gets notice that Gram's is having some changes—what changes I do not know. Nevertheless, the powers that be send her to a medical institution, the hospital, for some testing and medical care. She decides, for some reason, to get up out of bed in the middle of the night—probably to go to the toilet—while no one is around. She falls, hits her head and is dead within a couple of weeks.

.

The administration of hospitals in the past, as stated earlier in this piece, was usually allotted to the Church; volunteers would administer care. There was no money, *per se*, in it so the greedy need not apply, so to speak. The vocation of truly kind and caring people filled the roles of caregiver. Money and the corporate business world have changed all this. Money is the order of the day, and with it goes the scoundrel Sociopath who seeks their way toward self-fulfillment solely. From the top to the bottom, all, practically speaking, the truly caring people have left health care turned 'Healthcare' in refusal to sell their souls for mammon. We need them back in health care and healthcare. The void now that these true caregivers have left has been filled with the sociopaths of the day.

Another example: I had a patient (pt.) one day who was transferred from a skilled nursing facility (SNF; pronounced "sniff") for bleeding of her tracheotomy—a common admittance due to lack of trained personnel at these healthcare institutions. She, as most patients who come in with airway issues, whether needed or not, indicated or not, are

53

put on scheduled breathing treatments; billable therapy for which third parties pay? Nothing is for free!

So, sitting on the side of the bed, this pt. starts to talk right around the tracheostomy tube (trache), which is a pretty clear indication she is comfortable with the trache and has learned to manipulate it to her desires and needs.

[Communication is a huge issue for people with artificial airways. Not being able to communicate verbally has very deleterious effects in outcomes of the ill pt.]

We start talking, she and I, about the food—a common subject to talk about while standing around waiting for the unnecessary nebulized breathing treatment (tx) to finish.

[Nebulizer (often referred to as a "neb"): is a compressed gas-driven device for delivering a bronchodilator or other breathing medication via generating an aerosol that contains drug in saline solution. The nebulizer generates a cool mist and looks somewhat like a pipe, which the pt. puts in their mouth and breathes in the mist. Like smoking a pipe. Some patients like to call it "the peace pipe." Albuterol, at this time, was the most common bronchodilating drug used at this institution. These medications stimulate cardiac receptors with some patients, causing, in many cases, increased heart rates; newer medications have addressed some side effects, yet cardiac stimulation, among others, is still of concern when administering these drugs. Pronounced trembling with some patients' exposures to these drugs, especially in children is not uncommon. These nebulizer tx's usually run around five to 10 minutes depending on whether it is driven by an electric run compressor (which takes

54

considerably longer to completion) or medical gas driven (air or oxygen).]

[One has the liberty of turning up the gas flow to shorten 'neb' tx times when driven with a medical compressed gas—a cheap trick to "squeeze" in more treatments in less time, thereby increasing revenue without additional labor costs. Shortening tx times is a less effective tx, as most therapists know, yet do, seeing as most of these tx's seem to be ordered solely for the purpose of generating revenue and manipulating numbers and management calls for it. Very often these tx's do nothing positive, objectively, for the pt. At this institution all 'neb' tx's are run on 100% O2. Giving these tx's, with O2 is not doing any favors for the patients; delivering inappropriate medications and increasing reactive oxygen species (ROS's) exposure. But again, it is not about the pt. these days; it is about generating revenue. This needs to change; bring back patient-centered care.]

[Tachyphylaxis becomes a problem with inappropriate use of drugs; people build up a tolerance. Then when the drug is really necessary its efficacy is compromised requiring more of the drug to get the same effect. Eventually, in many cases, the drug stops having any positive effect.]

So this pt. I'm treating with the trache tells me she has been at the SNF for years and that they "only have two stars" for a rating score.

[Scale of one to five, five being the best]

"Do you want to know why they only have two stars?" She continues: "Because they are nasty over there. The help is rude and do not care. They do not care! They have no compassion for the patients."

"Any better here?" I ask.

"No, not really!

So there it is: the caregivers too have no compassion. They are going into medicine for the money, from top to bottom. It is a business, run by business people, who have very little to no idea what it is to work with sick people at the bedside. They only know the "bottom line." This needs to change. The "not-for-profit" is the joke played upon the community. The profit is just divvied up amongst management with bonuses and other such perks to show at the bottom-line that there is "no profit."

TRENDY ECONOMICS 101

Cutback, cutback, cutback! This is the "flavor-of-the-day" in the American field of business. Once a business starts a trend, it seems, everyone and his or her sister, and brother, wants to jump on the bandwagon. Now please know, it was not so long ago the medical initiations turned "healthcare" began to require all health care employees to refer to the patient as "customer" and then began pushing the old moniker: "the customer is always right," or more to the point: "give the customer what they want!"

The problem with this scenario is: what does the "customer"/patient know about current studies and advancements in medical treatments and technology (and how they can be skewed in biased directions, be it known, or unknown, unwittingly, or not)? Ignorance is bliss and it pays for some. For others the cost is very high.

We, most of us anyway, I dare say, have come to hear of, and know the term MRI as a medical tool in diagnostics, but do many know *what* the acronym stands for, or even what it does and how it works? Probably not; I'm not here to discuss the intricacies of magnetic resonance imaging and how it uses strong magnetic fields to create an image of tissues deep within the body by manipulating and viewing hydrogen atoms within (certainly this is a very overly simplified description of a technology way beyond the scope of this book).

What does the person who just became ill know about this new illness and strange turn of events in their own personal life? They might possibly have been heard saying, "I never, in a million years, dreamed I would find myself here." What about new medical technologies and modalities of treatments and medications that the medical profession is using to treat such illnesses in this modern-day, fast moving, ever-changing technological labyrinth? What would they know about such things? Very little, if anything at all, I suppose! So how can the patient-now-called-customer always be right? How? Many know nothing about their newly diagnosed illnesses, not to mention the best way to treat such illnesses. Fodder for fraud.

Another great irony of life is that many of the doctors of today do not know much about such things either. That is the scary part; at some point in our lives we must put our trust and faith in someone. And, as we all have probably heard at some point in our lives: "it is hard to find a good mechanic these days." When you do find one, invariably, many before you have come to the same conclusion and are so far ahead in the game that to get an appointment to see this practitioner is realistically way out of the realm of possibilities, for their reputation vastly precedes them (they made sure of it; marketing 101); for they are such a rare find in today's fast-paced deceptive world of fraudulent activities, robbing the system blind, by way of customer ignorance, that the latecomers must be turned away. Maybe a blessing in disguise!

One night in the medical/pulmonary ICU I get a call from the emergency room (ER) respiratory therapist that a 92-year-old male patient is coming up to the unit. He fell at home and hit his head. The family activated 911 emergency services that, upon arrival, intubated the somewhat unresponsive patient for airway protection and management.

The patient, after assessment in the trauma room, goes to the CT scanner to be scanned. Upon receiving a phone "report" from the ER therapist stating: "the patient is in the scanner now and we will be heading up to you as soon as he's done with the scan," I replied, "Great! Thanks! See you soon," thinking the scanning was done for the night and no travel for this patient; we can settle him in and make him comfortable and start active weaning to liberate the patient from the ventilator as soon as possible.

The patient arrives around 23:40 and is handed off to the ICU team. The transport team from the ER assures the ICU staff the patient just came from the CT scanner. The patient gets settled, and the doctors assess and write orders. One of the orders is for a stat (immediate) CT scan of the head. Now, again, the patient came to the hospital for a head injury, so it would be standard protocol to scan the head for any internal bleeding within the brain— evidence-based medicine—which, I probably do not have to add, a head bleed can be a very serious event requiring immediate attention. Time can be of great essence! The ordering doctor in the ICU is questioned as to the fact that the patient had a scan prior to admission into the unit.

[Unnecessary transports of critically ill pt. is not good pt care – pt transports in and of themselves are extremely dangerous on many levels, to say the least.]

The doctor says the head was not scanned. "Chest, abdomen, belly, and lower extremities were scanned but not the head," says the doc.

"Are you sure? Because the patient came to the hospital due to a fall, hitting his head!"

A call went down to the CT department where staff there confirmed: "the head was not done."

So back downstairs with this 92-year-old man at now 00:30, just into the next day. When we get down to CT scan I ask, "Why wasn't the head done when he was here an hour ago?" The CT technician tells me it was ordered initially but then canceled, and she says, "I don't know why."

In doing the math, it seems the "hospital," certainly aware of insurers questioning two CT scans in one day, "padding the bill," had found a way to extrapolate that extra revenue by playing the numbers game and getting a "two-for-one" CT scan paid for. The second scan was not on the same day. Bill for two when one would have been the better practice for the patient? There was no good reason in scanning this person, who fell and hit his head, and not scanning the head the first time around. But again: "the doctor knows best?" The hospital was able to bill, and presumably get paid, for two scans instead of one. Who is really calling the shots here? Who?

Of course my interpretation could be skewed and mistakes do happen, but this type of thing would happen much too frequently to pass off as coincidence and/or human error.

Now, you must understand, these CT scanners are very big technical and intricate machines that cost a great deal of money. The organization does not like to keep them idle. Idle does not pay the bills. So "order more CT scans please," we need the money—the unspoken (most of the time) word in the hallowed halls of the medical profession turned business enterprise to turn a profit. Don't be fooled by the "not-for-profit" mantra. Most will not speak out because they need the paycheck. The banker holding your mortgage doesn't care much for not getting their money. The banker doesn't care where you get your money, for the most part. They really only seem to care that they get theirs and that they get it on time. Otherwise, it's "out you go."

CORPERATE AMERICA

Fools we are for our desires.

Big business knows this and exploits it to the fullest—it is government set in place to tame these excessive desires of the unscrupulous. Yet government is not always able or willing to do this, for, after all, it is made up of humans. Our Founding 'Farmers' – I use "Farmers" for many of the Constitution Convention Delegates were in fact farmers of some sorts – were, I'm sure, well aware of the greedy desires of men and women and set in motion a new form of government. A government designed to keep such scoundrels at bay. The problem arises when the government climbs into bed with business, big business.

Great societies climb to lofty heights only on the backs of great statesmen and -women, stateswo/men who plant trees of which they themselves knew they would never enjoy the shade of which the saplings would bring. Many have tried and failed over the years. Greed seems to be a common denominator. Even ego is greed in a masked form. Corporate America, just like big government, takes a grand view and does not concern itself with trivial matters, such as the individuals like "you" and "me." "Numbers! Give us numbers. This is what we understand," they say.

Ignorance, however, seems only to invite fraud and advantaged abuses. Not always, but often, through the course of time, humans have been known to take advantage of the, shall we say, meek. This is, I like to think, why we have government in the first place: to keep people honest, to protect the 'little' from the 'big'. Government is the agency society puts in place to try to keep the unscrupulous honest; the bully at bay, an agency that has teeth to enforce the rules. It is an ongoing game jockeying for position to advance in the game of accumulating wealth. Some people do not like to play by the rules. Some do not like rules at all. Some manipulate rules and laws in their favor. These are the people who are always calling for the removal of regulations and "let the free market function as it should: freely." The problem with the free market philosophy is, when you have everyone in it for himself or herself, the individual becomes obsessed with the competition (the Jones' effect) and begins to lose sight of the bigger picture of community and how we are all in this life together.

So to turn a business into a money-making machine for the sole sake of acquiring massive amounts of 'wealth' benefits no one but the ones who worship mammon. Yet we are taught, some of us anyway, that one cannot worship mammon and God at the same time. So if God is love, then the love of money must be some perverted adulteration of the concept of love, and the one who goes after money and material things, for the inflation of "thy-self's" ego and pride, is only deluding themselves into the illusion of buying happiness.

Do we all not already know that money cannot buy happiness? I'll bet most of us feel we certainly would like to find out firsthand, for ourselves whether money can or cannot buy true happiness. Semantics? Maybe. Some may refer to us as: "Thomases."

The corporate insurance companies want documentation that a modality or medication works before they will pay. Fair enough. The rub comes when the ones who want to be paid are the ones producing the studies that show a medical procedure or medication works. The doctors within the institutions to be paid are the ones conducting the studies that "show" "objective" truths to the effect. Many studies are deliberately skewed to lean toward desired results. Some covertly more than others, and some may be not at all skewed. Yet again: it is impossible to really know what might have been; what lay ahead on the path not taken. What works on some does not necessarily work on another for reasons, many times, unknown. I've heard some people say caffeine puts them to sleep.

Did Henry Ford pay his workers a wage geared toward the purchase of his wares? Does not the "free-market" capitalist economy thrive on created markets? Is this really a "free" market where producers competitively pedal their wares? Or have these corporations become, as my mother liked to say: "too big for their britches?"

Now, don't get me wrong, as I have stated previously, there have been some great "goods" that have advanced greatly the human experience of life in a more healthy and positive manner. But, for the most part, the moneyed class (venture capitalists) learned a long time ago that marketing is the name of the game, and the new wave hospital executive is all about creating the market via advertising. Look around the cities of the U.S. these days as you drive along the highways and byways: billboards manipulatively touting the impression that their local hospitals are the place to go with any type of concern or questions about health. These billboards may say things like: "Among the top ten best rated hospitals in the country" or "The best neonatal/pediatric care on the East Coast." The question arises as to who is doing the rating? When one looks at an online independent review platform, like Google or, say, Yelp, one finds a whole different story. Scrolling down and getting past some of the fiction that the companies themselves put up to help improve their ratings, you can get a pretty good idea that something is amiss. Objectively, however, one can read between the lines and get a pretty good idea as to what really may be going on at these institutions. Even at that, most have no idea what really goes on behind the curtain.

Here is a notion to ponder going into the next chapter: third parties usually will not pay unless there is "well-founded" objective evidence that shows a particular medical device, medication, or procedure has a very good success rate.

STUDY FOR FUNDS

I remember talking with parents of patients with cystic fibrosis (CF) about how insurance companies would not pay for "The Vest," an automated percussive/vibration device for chest physiotherapy. Chest physical therapy (CPT) is a big part of these patients' lives, daily lives, FOR LIFE! To do this manually is a lot of work for the one providing the percussions and vibrations; automation, for parents and their children, is a Godsend. Technology does have its place in medicine. Nevertheless, I remember hearing the parents complain for a number of years that insurance would not pay. Then, I suppose with enough gathered documented information over time showing positive results, the insurance companies had enough objective documentation as to the effectiveness of The Vest that they began to pay. Which segues right into my question: who is putting out these studies that convince the insurance companies to pay for a procedure or treatment of some sort? The medical profession most often, that's who—the ones who are, by the by, doing the billing in many of these instances. Now in the case of The Vest there is strong evidence that it produces positive results.

However, being involved, just by way of working in the live laboratory, the ICU, I, many times, have, in all probability, been part of later published studies. Many times this "blindness" is crucial for many reasons, not least of which is that the unprofessionalism and incompetence that abounds in the medical profession and hospital institutions can seriously skew results. And, on the other end of the spectrum, even in double-blinded studies, physicians can, and do, "weight," shall we say, results in their own favor.

Now we get into the gray area of conflicting interests. It is no wonder when a new procedure, or even an older elective procedure, say cardiac surgery, involves some pretty extensive screening of patients before they are selected as a candidate for the procedure. This is to "insure" (pun intended) the success of the numbers game at the third-party's "players" table. Only qualified prospective candidates for the procedure, the patients that the medical team feels will have the most likelihood of a successful outcome, will be accepted. This is to insure good numbers for the institution but also for the team and individual physician alike, for, with a high success rate, they will, by review, attract more patients and exact more revenue for the guaranty. Certainly it is a lot less expensive if a procedure goes as planned, from an insurer's point of view, than the expense of remedial measures if not. A numbers game nevertheless.

This is where accounting comes in: the manipulation of numbers. Healthcare today is a numbers game, and, cynically, I have often thought, business 101 has become a requirement in medical school these days. The third-party payers and even drug companies desire and maybe even require it.

Marketing and accounting drive the industry of healthcare today. Let's take a closer look.

Let me give you a "hypothetical" situation where one might believe something had been done when if fact it had not, like, say, in a meta-analysis.

At some point a young, big, burly, otherwise healthy adult male person in about his 30s is found down in a snow bank just outside a local barroom during the wee hours of a frigidly cold January morning. This report came to the ICU along with the patient: a friend who had gone to the bar with him, the patient, that night, last saw him at some time in the evening "going outside for a smoke"—being Massachusetts and no smoking inside public places.

Upon leaving the bar at closing, or at some point in the night, the friend looks for his buddy who had gone out for the smoke and finds him face-down in a snow bank: unresponsive, stiff, and with very shallow or maybe even absent breathing—EtOH can distort one's view of a situation. Emergency Medical Services (EMS) is activated and intubate the subject upon arrival. CPR is initiated and continued on and off en route to the ER, then x-rays, CT scan, and up to the ICU. He was assessed and cleaned up at the same time.

[It is amazing to watch some of these ICU nurses and aides. When a patient comes in, they swarm, like bees or ants, all at once on the patient. Everyone has their place; they flip, in this case, him, the patient from side to side while quickly cleaning the backside and assessing for anything unusual and making note. The patient is "spick-and-spanned," to use a phrase, in a matter of minutes, smelling-like-a-rose. I'm not kidding; I have seen, no exaggeration, patients weighing over 300 pounds, who, upon going into respiratory failure, due to a restrictive pulmonary derangement called "fat," activate EMS because of shortness of breath (SOB): dyspnea. The person is so large it was said they had to take down a wall to get him out of the house; he had not been out of his recliner for so many years family could not say how long. He would urinate and defecate in the chair. Boy did he stink when he came up to the unit. Those nurses and aides flipped this guy around, scrubbed, and probably had to pick a little, or more, and had him cleaned up like never before in no time at all. When his family was allowed in to see him, they at first thought they were in the wrong room; they had never, in very long memory, seen him so clean:

shaven, hair cleaned by "shampoo-in-a-can," combed and neat—like a new man. Impressive.]

Anyway, I digress, back to our "abominable snowman" patient found in the snow bank. He is difficult to oxygenate, but otherwise drugs have, for the time being, satisfied the electrical impulse desires of his heart muscle to continue rhythmic contractions.

The doctors order epoprostenol—a strong and toxic vasodilator that can be given intravenously, or inhaled, to dilate the pulmonary artery, allowing greater blood flow to the lungs and therefore greater chance for oxygenation of the blood to transport it, the O2, to the tissue—to be given via aerosol (inhaled). This is to be done through the ventilator/patient circuitry using two IV pumps. One is used to pump saline and the other epoprostenol into an upstream positioned mesh nebulizer in the ventilator circuit, both set at the doctor-ordered rate and concentration based on body mass indexing.

The respiratory therapist on this night was the one who knows everything (I'm sure you know the type, where incompetence abounds and without the least bit of their own knowledge of such a thing. It would be funny if it wasn't so scary and sad) and will always be there to save the day and take the credit when things are going good, but when things start going south the first one to start pointing the finger in any direction but their own. This therapist sets the epoprostenol pump to a level where it is not pumping the epoprostenol at all, as would come to be found out eight hours later at shift change when the oncoming therapist notices the epoprostenol bag had not emptied at all.

To the point: it was documented that the drug was given when it was not. The record may show an attempt at epoprostenol rescue when in fact it was not. The record remains unchanged, I imagine. A meta-analysis of medical records would be giving erroneous information. This is just one scenario of many where human error played a role. This is true in many, many cases. In the medical profession there is much incompetence, just like all large institutions I suppose; yet one thing medical professionals are very competent in is covering their tracks.

It is easy to push numbers around and even easier to lie. Some people seem to be without scruples, ethics, or shame—no conscience. The medical profession likes numbers and likes to manipulate them to their fancy, as I have said. I'll give you another example of this.

In the Respiratory Care Department a budget needs to be justified, and it is not easy to quantify every little task that a therapist might perform through the course of a 12-hour shift. Things come up. Nurses on the floor may pull a therapist aside knowing the breadth of knowledge some well-trained and seasoned practitioners have in their lab coat or under their belt, if you like. A nurse may ask, "Could you just poke your head in and take a look at my patient? See what you think. They seem a little off from last night." "Sure." Now this patient is not on respiratory services and has no orders, so there really is no billing involved. But there is time involved. Certainly to assess a patient well, as the nurse in this case is asking the therapist to do, takes some time. If the patient is unknown to the therapist, the first place to go if there is time, is the medical chart and get some background information about the patient. Certainly some information, no doubt, will be ascertained from the nurse, like age, gender, reason for visit, diagnosis, history, length of stay, oxygen requirements, cause of nurse's concern, any diagnostic testing results, and the like. Then to the physical assessment; seasoned therapists can tell a lot just by looking at a person: obese or frail or emaciated; older looking than age; skin pigmentation tells a tale; chest girth, shape, and excursion; any audible breath sounds; breathing pattern; body language like grimacing from pain; sitting up in bed, or on the side of the bed, or lying in the bed on one side or another, upright (Fowlers position), semi-Fowlers, or flat, are the tips of the fingers blue or clubbed, are the ankles and feet edematous. A quick walk-in assessment gives the therapist a novel of information about the subject at hand. This becomes an involuntary instant assessment trait on many therapists' part of all living beings encountered, as vocation has its say whether agreed with or not; always assessing.

After introductions, and capacity, the therapist will ask if they, the patient, are so-and-so, using the first name only. If they say "yes," will then ask them to state their last name and date of birth. One gets a lot of information just from this brief encounter; however, it does take time, and patients do not like staff running into and out of their rooms when they are ill and in a strange place and don't really know what is going on. It is a great cause for concern, and it can create great anxiety for patients—I don't like it when I find myself on that side of the bed, meaning *in it*, as a patient.

So just by getting the patient to talk the therapist can see if the patient is truly short of breath. If some patient starts by saying: "I'm short of breath" and then begins telling their whole life's story from start to finish without the therapist getting a word in edgewise, they know this patient is not short of breath. If they were, they would, in no way, be talking in full sentences. They would be gasping for breaths in-between one or two words, maybe three. Their lips would be bluish-gray, cyanotic, and most likely pursed.

More to the point: time is involved, but nothing is billable for respiratory services—the nurse, and patient, appreciated it, though. This concern of the nurse for their patient is valid and appropriate. What might be found after a partially complete on-the-spot assessment is that the patient is "wet," meaning: fluid in the lungs causing an increase in their work-of-breathing (WOB or IWB) due to a lack of accessible alveoli, for the air sacs of the lung are so full of interstitial fluid that there is no surface exposed for gas exchange. Gravity plays a role, and when the patient sits up the fluid goes to the bases of the lungs, giving the patient some relief. This is where auscultation would reveal fine inspiratory crackles within the bases of the lungs, which can be indicative of fluid buildup. The further up the lung fields the crackles are heard, the more fluid in the lungs and the more sensation of dyspnea the patient feels. The O2 level decreases to a critical level as the CO2 eventually rises, putting the patient in a compromising hypoxic and acidotic state, and, when the hyperventilation stops due to fatigue, hypercarbic respiratory failure ensues.

"Call the doctor about a chest x-ray and ask them about some diuretic."

Time with no billable charge for Respiratory services, yet life saving for the patient. Should the nurse have known this? Yes! And most likely did but concurrence can go a long way in getting the doctor out of bed and do something. So the Respiratory Department is looking for ways to document what they do so as to justify the funding of a budget. This certainly makes sense, to a point, but some services that save lives are not so easily defined. In this Respiratory Department therapists had been, for some time, complaining that the billing codes were not descript enough to reflect some of these services that are provided to the hospital population yet are "unbillable." The director and management along with some overly zealous staff members, perhaps, redefined the billing codes to try to capture all that a therapist might attend to in the course of a 12-hour shift. The codes can be general in scope to at least give some concept of time if not product provided by the therapist. The codes were changed. After a short period of time the director sends out an e-mail asking all therapist to go back to the original coding for "RT" time because, with the new system, the "numbers are much lower" than before and will have a deleterious effect of the overall view of productivity. So, in reality, the director of respiratory services is asking her staff to "fudge" numbers to make the department look, on paper, a certain way. Is this patient-centered care? No it is not! But it looks good on paper from a study standpoint.

And, when going to upper management, who only seem to focus on numbers and the bottom line— no matter how much they tell you they care about the patients—the numbers warrant a certain number of FTEs (full time equivalent or employee, if you like) to run the department. Now this all makes good-sensed business practice in my estimation, but for the fact that in the real world, when one finds oneself in the trenches of survival, things can be a whole lot different as to how it plays out. It is wise to know what goes on in the inner-workings of any business; in healthcare one sometimes gets the impression, to use another phrase, that "the left hand doesn't know what the right hand is doing." or, more realistically, having heard it ring throughout the hallways of the hospital: "There is a disconnect between management and staff." But, can these highly educated people be so stupid? One would have to come to the most logical answer as: NO. Is this all by design? Business practice—to keep expenses low and revenue steady, what the free-market capitalists like to call: "what the market will bear."

Many times things will get done at the bedsides that are not part and parcel for a particular study that might be in play. Or even data tapped at a later date for a base in a meta-analysis. Nurses want their patients to get better, and they want the numbers to show this objectively to the medical staff.

If a nurse is struggling with a very sick, intubated and mechanically ventilated patient, and the saturation of oxygen in the blood (SaO2 or "sats") drop, say from the necessary turning of a patient to prevent a decubitus ulcer (skin breakdown or "bed sores") from developing, the nurse, very often, will call for the respiratory therapist to come to the bedside and "fix them," meaning increase the patient's oxygenation numbers. The therapist might first suction any secretions out of the airway and, in usually a futile attempt with the equipment available, the lungs too. Generally, in this institution, O2, which is classified as a drug, needs a doctor's order to be administered or discontinued or changed in any direction in relation to an increase or decrease from current levels of FiO2. It is common practice, however, and the ventilators have a special "100% O2 suction" button to be depressed for suctioning of the patient that administers via the ventilator 100% O2 for two to three minutes to "hyper-oxygenate" the patient prior to and during the suctioning of the endotracheal (ET) tube aka: artificial airway or "breathing tube." This procedure, for obvious reasons, will, in most cases, increase the blood/oxygen saturation pretty well if the lung parenchyma (working parts of an organ; in this case the lungs) is at all functioning, even if not at total capacity. But this is really just a Band-Aid, for once all those newly introduced O2 molecules get metabolized, the blood saturation drops again. Not always, but often. Sometimes it is just a matter of the patient settling down again and the fluid in the lungs being redistributed by gravity and other alveoli getting re-recruited to allow for gas exchange. With Acute Respiratory Distress Syndrome (ARDS) patients this does not often happen, and more aggressive measures may be needed to increase blood/oxygen levels and sustain them for any period of time. One bedside maneuver taken in these situations is what many like to call a "recruitment maneuver." All this really is, is having the ventilator give a breath at a set tidal volume (Vt) and hold it for a certain amount of time at a certain pressure. What this does is helps "pop" open some of the alveoli that may have collapsed (flattened) or may be filled with fluid and allows for more stretching of the surface wall area to be exposed to gas – not necessarily a good thing, more like a last ditch effort. Different institutions, or doctors, may use different pressures and times for these maneuvers, but in this institution at the time it was "30 for 30," meaning a pressure of 30 cm H2O for 30 seconds, repeating three times in succession if necessary. It is remarkable in many cases the good effect one can achieve with these pulmonary compromised patients. Yet just as often it is only a quick fix; a temporary stay; or, as I like to say: just "a Band-Aid." It can occasionally buy some desperately needed time, giving the lungs time to heal but, all in all, may do more harm than good, for no study has shown a change in morbidity from recruitment maneuvers.

I'll tell you why: human error can be a huge factor of which many may never know. As I have said, the medical profession has, at the very least, become very competent in hiding the truth.

One night, working the infamous "torture chamber": 6 ICU, the respiratory therapist working in the unit for the night had a "difficult-to-oxygenate" pulmonary pt. This patient was intubated and being mechanically ventilated.

Another therapist on their way into the unit to help out if needed saw right away upon entering the unit that just about all the nurses and the two doctors of the unit are surrounding the patient's bed.

The two night doctors are there at the foot of the bed and the acting respiratory therapist was next to the bed on the opposite side of the ventilator.

[It is very unwise for the therapist to be on the opposite side of the bed from where the ventilator is in case something needs to be addressed emergently with the ventilator and the interface to the pt.—you will get a glimpse of what I am talking about in a minute.]

As the second therapist walks into the unit, one of the doctors steps over to him and quietly says something to the effect: "I think we have a pneumo!" (Pressure pneumothorax = collapsed lung; emergently deadly) This patient was about to die! Hypertensive along the extreme, tachycardic (rapid heart rate) and tachypnic (rapid respirations) and becoming more and more difficult to ventilate; peak inspiratory pressures were high and if the lung wasn't blown (which it was not) it was about to. Clearly the patient was in great distress. As the entering therapist walked over to the foot of the bed to get a better look at the patient, the monitors and numbers, he quickly assessed that the positive end-expiratory pressure (Peep) on the ventilator was set at a very high 30 cm H2O p.

"She's on 30 of Peep?" the therapist inquires. At which point the doctor, the one who questioned about the potential "pneumo," springs into action, lunges at the ventilator within a fraction of a second, and turns the Peep down to a more manageable level. Then a voice from above rings out: "That'll do it!" This was EICU.

[EICU is an electronic system monitoring all of the ICU beds via cameras and audio. The Attending Physicians manning the "command post"—at a remote location—can see the patients and all monitors and numbers, in real time, in all ICUs throughout all the institution's campuses. These serve as an aid to the "physicians-in-training" who are on-site at night in the ICUs to help in consulting an attending physician toward the making of good diagnoses and decisions (in theory).]

The therapist this night, as I had said, was on the wrong side of the bed and, with all the other staff mulling around the bed, rendered useless. Unless, of course, he reached for the ET tube and disconnected the pt. from the ventilator to create a leak and relieve the excess pressure, but this would have caused its own set of problems with de-recruitment of the patient's lungs.

This patient's life was saved by the therapist's quick and accurate assessment of the emergent situation and the fast acting physician to turn down the Peep. This quick thinking therapist became a small-time "guru" for a short time, as word got around, by his quick diagnosis that saved the patient's life, of which the whole rest of the ICU team, and the attending physician in "the box," had missed. After this incident word must have gone around and many of the new intern doctors just out of medical school would seek out this therapist and ask to teach them about mechanical ventilation.

In the end it was found that this therapist (on the wrong side of the bed) performed a recruitment maneuver on this patient to help with oxygenation, (without a doctor's order) and had forgotten to turn the pressure back down after 30 seconds. This caused an excessively large increase in intra-thoracic pressures for a prolonged period of time via the expanded pressurized lungs, at 30 cm H_2O p., pushing on other organs; the heart was not happy. The Attending Physician in "the box" was, shall we say, humbled? The respiratory therapist on the wrong side of the bed lost his job. Human error—

which, I'm pretty sure, the medical record does not reflect the incident.

There are many other examples of a more directed nature in promoting good results from a procedure for numbers purposes to show a medical procedure or technique works when in fact it is questionable. Such as proning a pt, when there is not an oxygenation issue with the patient in the first place that would warrant proning.

[Proning of a patient: placing them face down in the bed. This is done to utilize more posterior aspects of lung parechyma that might otherwise be found atelectatic (collapsed or flattened alveoli/small air sacs within the lung) while artificially ventilating in an attempt to improve oxygenation. Newer bed units allow for flipping the whole bed with the pt strapped tightly in.]

Proning is a very dangerous technique due to the intricacies of flipping a sick and compromised patient with many lines and tubes hanging out: easy targets to be kinked or snagged and/or displaced accidentally. Proning beds today are very specific pieces of medical equipment where a patient is strapped securely in the bed, as said. Strapping is tightly arranged over the chest and abdomen, arms and legs, and head to keep the pt securely in the bed while it is flipped upside-down itself with the patient in it. These straps securing the patient are very restrictive, as one might imagine, severely restricting the natural and necessary excursions of the chest during spontaneous, or otherwise, respirations. There have been cases where objectivity was manipulated by tightening the chest straps creating an oxygen deficiency via chest restriction. The attending physician ordering the proning, which now comes off as "successful," has the numbers to show success when in fact, there really was no physiological reason for the desaturation other than intended externally physically induced hypoxemia resulting in hypoxia. Thus creating a real danger to the patient yet looked good for the doctor who takes credit for saving a life. And of course bills the 'third-party' for it. The doctor did not like it when the nurses called Respiratory to address the problematic oxygenation issue while in the throws of proning and all the therapist had to do was release the straps of the chest and oxygenation shot up to 100%. This made the objectivity of the study look bad. "Put the straps back on and flip her. *QUICKLY!* Before Respiratory comes back." A successful case of proning; saved this patient's life; stretching the imagination for outcome and income, all the while really just 'artificially-restricting' the pt from breathing.

Too many times patient's are tortured with unnecessary treatments to insure revenue for the institution.

PLACEBO EFFECT

The placebo effect has proved tried and true on many levels and occasions. Yet in today's medical profession, like many other professions of today, transparency is the call to order, all the while the realities of the cause are cloaked and blinded. Fear being the tool used to motivate.

Transparency is good, but maybe not in all cases. As we know children need time to mature mentally before they are capable of handling complex issues of the real world like darkness. And it is also true that some people get stuck in ruts.

However, if a medical professional, for instance, tells a patient that there is no physiological reason for their dyspnea they usually are in disbelief. Hypothetically if told: "I have a pill here that will cure your ills," the placebo effect can and very often does greatly diminish the anxiety induced dyspnea and relieves the symptoms associated with the SOB, for, as the American Lung Association likes to say, "When you can't breathe, nothing else matters." Yet, if the patient is told the truth: "this is just a sugar pill, but if you truly believe it will help, it could."— chances are it may, for a while. Maybe, but probably not!

Today, unfortunately, the placebo effect has been adulterated to increase revenues to profits. The only problem with this scenario is that the patient is not the one to profit, and the placebo is not always sugar coated.

Here is an example: one of the directors of the Respiratory Care Department where I worked would argue that giving a breathing treatment to a patient who is experiencing a bout of SOB is good policy, even if physiologically there is no objectifiable indication for the SOB. But psychologically there are.

So, management would say, "just give the neb." Even though the patient was not bronchoconstricted and the medication would have no positive effect. In this institution of which I speak all neb tx's are given with 100% O2 – the driving gas – along with Albuterol as the bronchodilator. A quick burst of energy to the pt from the increased O2. In the long run however this is deleterious to the patients overall good health: oxygen toxicity. Damage to and remodeling of lung tissue on a molecular level: pulmonary fibrosis.

This director would say: "just give them the neb. Sometimes it makes them feel better just to be smoking something." When explained to this director that, in that line of thinking, we could be giving a placebo, like normal saline (NaCl), and have the same effect. She fell silent and could not disagree.

The policy stands however: give rescue-breathing medications if someone feels they are having a hard time breathing regardless of objectivity. Poor medicine at best; poor judgment to say the least! Now I agree a one-time tx to assess is not bad practice but to continue with no positive effect is not good medicine.

[There are times when the sound of wheezing is a relief for it indicates there is some air movement within the lungs. When a true asthmatic's lungs shut down these patients struggle severely just to move any air. When they do begin to "open up," wheezing is the indication that air is beginning to move. This objectivity is real and a relief to all concerned in these cases. A breath of fresh air, if you will! In subjective cases not so much.]

Nevertheless, as I continue to say in regards to anxiety: "There are better medications out there." But the nebulizers cost less than anxiety medications. Giving bronchodilating medications when not indicated is a great disservice to the patients, and the community, as we begin to see more and more of these patients developing tracheobronchomalacia (TBM): airways losing tone. When the doctors cannot find the cause of a problem with their patients, they have a fancy medical term they like to use: "idiopathic." But, really, who is the idiot? And who is pathetic? And once again we begin to see the inner workings of an institutional moneymaking-machine culture.

The licensed medical "professionals" are medicating people unnecessarily. And for what: revenue and numbers?

Fear is a strong motivating factor on many levels for many.

[Side-effects of over and inappropriate use of bronchodilators can cause lose of muscle and structure tone. TBM: loss of tone of the bronchial and tracheal cartilages, muscles, and connective tissues, can be debilitating. An observation noted over many years of such unnecessary tx's: the trachea and smaller airways lose tone and thus ability to stay patent. The airways now collapse in on themselves, causing difficulty in moving air out of the lungs. Wheezing ensues: a high-pitched musical sound generated from within the chest cavity by forcing gas through narrowed lumina.]

When a doctor now hears wheezing, s/he thinks of bronchial constriction and, you guessed it, orders more bronchodilatory medications to be given at a closer frequency. This very often gives no relief, for they are not constricted, they are restricted. Doctors don't get it, or they do not want to get it, because what they are really doing is ensuring their patient base for years to come. At some point these patients will need to be intubated and ventilated, then eventually "trached," which now bypasses the upper airway structures thereby reducing airway resistance to the lung parenchyma by way of reduction in length. At some point it might be suggested to have the trachea replaced. Now the surgeon is involved in the "saving" of this patient's life. The patient, putting their faith in the doctor—for "the doctor knows best"—now is so thankful to the medical profession for saving their lives, when in fact this is iatrogenic!

I'll give you an example of another side of the same coin. In the ICU, when working toward liberating a patient from a ventilator (breathing machine), a patient who has demonstrated the strength, willingness, cognition, and mentation appropriate for extubation (removal of the "breathing tube") sometimes will quickly fail a "spontaneous breathing trial" (SBT) due to anxiety. Telling the patient "we are going to have you breathe on your own right now" can send them into immediate bouts of respiratory distress due to fear and anxiety; fear of the unknown; fear of death. After all, it is this breathing machine that just saved their lives and has been keeping them breathing and alive.

When you can't breathe nothing else matters. The sensation of impending doom is a strong motivator for survival mode. If someone has become accustomed to something else doing the breathing for him or her, they might, and are, hesitant to have that "security-blanket," "the breathing machine," taken away. In their eyes it is a life and death situation. And why not, for, whatever the situation that brought them to the ICU—very often COPD in these circumstances—was a life-threatening event, such as acute respiratory failure; many times acute-on-chronic. They could not effectively breathe on their own, and doom was, in fact, impending and imminent

82

without medical intervention. For better or worse, who wouldn't be scared? So anxiety is the barrier to a successful weaning trial many, many times.

Tachypnea can be a sign and symptom of many things, one of which is anxiety, as I've already mentioned. It is an ineffectual way to breathe, causing, in many instances, a failure of a breathing trial geared toward liberating the patient from the ventilator. But—and I've had patients themselves indicate to me—if the trial is begun without informing them they are about to "do all the breathing on their own" while still connected to the ventilator, they pass the test, many times, without a hitch, followed by, within a two-hour window, a successful extubation. I have seen, time and time again, patients fail weaning trials due to the fear of breathing on their own—even when all indications are they can, and do, once the fear is relieved. So more often than not a physician will treat this with pharma-chemical products; this works, but now you have sedative chemicals on board of which the body must metabolize, and these are patients, very often, with multiple systems weakened by illness that have a hard time processing/metabolizing drugs. The work required to metabolize anything is going to consume oxygen. This is oxygen the patient could use in other aspects of the healing process. We give supplemental O2, but now you run the risk of oxygen free radicals or ROS, and the havoc they can play at the molecular level. The "placebo effect" works. It is funny with some of these patients. They ask you not to tell them when the breathing trial is to begin. You don't; they do well. Then, you go in the room and say, "Hey, you've been breathing on your own now for two hours, and you're doing great!" They become tachypnic; their Vt plummet, resulting in a blood/oxygen desaturation and now a failed weaning trial. Sometimes silence is golden. Sometimes it is a rapid wean and you "just pull the tube," like ripping off a Band-Aide: one quick motion and out. And the patient is happy.

On other fronts, patients might be complaining of SOB for reasons that have nothing to do with breathing at all. But they don't know that; they only know they "can't catch my breath; my chest is heavy." ANXIETY! And who would not be anxious. You're sick enough to be in the hospital (at least that is what the doctor tells you); you are in a strange place in a strange bed, surrounded by strangers. Many come into the room swiftly, unannounced; poke and prod then, just as abruptly as they came, leave. Who would not be anxious? So they are having a hard time breathing. Who wouldn't?

"Take a deep breath; in through your nose and out through your mouth" I will tell them. Quietly telling them to: "relax, you're all right! Take a big breath in and hold it for a count of 10." I tell them to "purse-lip breathe," which is pursing your lips together, like you are going to whistle, and exhaling slowly out, to slow the breathing and allow time for gases to exchange in the lungs—O_2 perfuse into and CO_2 out of the blood—and, at the same time, creates some "back pressure" in the lungs and airways to help in preventing prolapse of the airways. Pulmonary patients' diseased lungs enhance their sensation of dyspnea, along with the sensation of impending doom. Hate that impending doom.

So a little bit of coaching, on a very simple technique that almost anyone can master, immediately results in real-time actual relief for many of these patients—a vast majority. I will have patients watch their saturation monitor and see the oxygen percentage rise considerably, in real time, right as they are doing it. I have even been able to turn down supplemental oxygen (and all those ROS's that go along with it) and still watch the oxygen saturation rise while performing these deep-breathing exercises. Very impressive, even to doctors who, very often, do not seem to understand the concept of physiologic human biology. They have been trained in pharmacology. That is where the money is. The "placebo effect," however, has its place. Transparency can, at times, be a blocker of placebo. What to do, what to do? Objectively we must look at subjectivity. Pulmonary rehabilitation through way of education goes a long way. Just not as much money in it, I suppose. The modality today to get the patient to commit to treatment is fear. It works; sad but true. Business uses this to advance their profit base.

SUBJECTIVITY vs. OBJECTIVITY

Today we practice evidence-based medicine.
Or do we?

Today we know that many physicians have been handing out narcotics like candy—per doctor's order. This has its pitfalls and ramifications and has come to be a major problem within our communities and society at large. Doctors have made addicts out of good, upstanding, productive members of our society—ruined many good people's productive lives. Innocently? Maybe. Yet, as I will show in this discourse, money has played a huge role in the ever-evolving profession of medicine.

Subjectivity verses objectivity. Is all this out of ignorance or by design, toward revenue generation? In today's medical profession here in the U.S. it is all about the money. This is the theme of this book. Business trumps medicine in a venture capitalistic-driven free-market society. Most doctors that I've dealt with over the years do not really seem to care about the patient. They care about billing. Some of the doctors that truly do care have left their practice years ago. Many of the people who go into medicine, in this U.S. of A., these days, are all about ego and money.

The medical profession is making us sick, and making money, profits off of it. This is by design. Not until the money is gone do they let a patient die. If there is still money in the patient's account the patient is kept alive until the institution has extracted as much of this money as possible. More often than not the patient is subjected to treatments and testings they do not want, or debatably, need, before they are allowed to die. Much like lawyers: many seem your best friend until the money is gone, then they don't know who you are. ER doctors have been heard complaining that they have been reprimanded "for not ordering enough CT scans."

It is pretty well known by now that many sick elderly people just want to die peacefully at home, but the doctor just won't let them. The law sometimes, many times, comes down hard on people who do not seek medical advice when an illness sets in. Unless, of course, the patient signs out against medical advice (AMA), and then, if the patient does sign the document to be discharged from the hospital against medical advice, the patient is cut off from all future medical treatments and therapies. Even on a home or outpatient basis, such as physical therapy, which is a well-known "tried and true" modality of treatment for many. The patient is "blackballed" or "blacklisted" as "non-compliant" and denied third-party payment to treat. Many, putting their faith in the doctor, believe if the doctor says it is true, it must be. And even then, one more MRI, one more CT scan, before they pull the plug. The medical school seems to have dropped the ethics class and replaced it with financial planning. Subjectively they spout objectivity towards final release, yet many, many times it is really toward increasing revenue for the institution.

Marketing is the order of the day. Tell them enough times the yellow shirt is blue, and they will come to believe it. Tell them to come for a cure, and they will come. But, you must play by their rules or you will not be allowed to play at all. This is why I like "health-maintenance" organizations: it is best to take care of yourself, stay healthy, and stay away from the doctor. Once the medical professionals have you in their systematic grips, they are hell-bent on keeping you there until the coffers have been completely "letted" of all potential resource, be it house and home or retirement accounts. The medical industry seems to be out to rule the world by any means possible be it by hook or by crook.

How many times of late have the courts taken a child away from parents because the parents did not want the suggested medical treatment for their child? Many! Take a Boston hospital, for instance. A very publicized case ensued in the 90's (maybe later) when the hospital refused the parents their child; who was not allowed to go home at the parents' request because the medical professionals did not think it in the best interest of the child. Who's in charge here? Institutions seem to be. In many cases this is not a bad thing but when business obfuscates ones view to deceive for profits sake the patients and their families suffer unnecessarily.

In this country, in this day and age, if we do not follow along with the status quo, we are labeled as mentally unfit, or worse, and, you guessed it, institutionalized. We are being sold a bill-of-goods. We now, by statute, are required to support this "machine" or face sanctions. Every citizen is required by law to pay into the health insurers coffers. The only way out is by defection: denouncing citizenship and moving to another country. We have outlived our ability to pay, so society's future has been bankrupted—billed as the savior of the world when in fact we are billed to fund the venture capitalist, who, by the by, are the ones deciding for us where our hard-earned surplus is sequestered for their own personal use. You know who really gets the best health care, don't you? The people with the money to pay for it! Many times within the hospital one is told by management "that is so and so's sister," or brother, "take good care of them." "What are you saying? I have to give different grades of care depending on who the patient is?"

SURPLUS

Life is one big lesson in letting go.

Surplus: the beginning of warring and destruction; how much surplus produced by ingenuity has been squandered away by destructive warring? Why are people working so hard chasing the carrot when others take the best produce and just keep waving that illusive carrot in front of our faces, keeping us moving forward to the institutions design, yet which we the underlings are never to attain?

Coming out of Cambodia are stories of Western technologies being introduced into the farming community back sometime in the 80s about the benefits of fertilizing their rice crops. Westerners promoted and supplied the new fertilizers to local Khmer farmers to "double" the Cambodian rice yields. Left them with the supplies, know-how, and means to double their crops yield in one year's time.

The Westerners said, "We will be back next year to see how it all worked out for you."

"Ok, see you next year at harvest time."

The following year the technocrat-capitalists came back to see how the progress was. Expecting a boon in crop harvest, these technically advanced corporations, promoting the use of fertilizers, herbicides, and pesticides, were surprised at what they came back to find: the local farmers had only planted half their lot and produced the same amount as the prior year's harvest. They only produced what they would need for one year; having no use for surplus, they had no interest in long-term storage. The westerners were dumbfounded.

"Why did you not plant all your fields?" they asked.

"We only grow what we need," was the reply.

Surplus: the beginning of strife between the "haves" and the "have-nots"! What to do with surplus?

What to do with surplus if and/or when we might find ourselves with some? In this modern-day era, many will put surplus away for a "rainy day," such as "retirement," for example. In this new nuclear age, where families are small and demands are high, many do not have the time or initiative to care for the elderly, who are thus "institutionalized"; to be cared for in their "golden" years, placed in "a home." Paid for via those "coffers" set up years ago and funded in various sorts of ways to pay for the elders' care. Family members of today are too much at the "grind," trying desperately to "squirrel away" some of their own surplus (if there is any) for the day when it is their turn to be cared for in an institution. Families these days seem too busy in their never-ending hustle-bustle lives trying to keep up with the demands this society puts on its inhabitants in this, what some like to call, never-ending-cycle of life. Or so it might appear.

Nevertheless, the money – the voucher to stores -- is supposed to be there "when the time comes." So, many people who have the luxury of being "gainfully" employed have to make decisions on what to do with the excess. Many will put money aside for these "golden" years to be able to provide for themselves and try, as much as possible, to avert the old-age institution where care is lacking and elder abuse is prevalent—a problem very often just swept under the carpet. This is nothing new, people are so wrapped up in their own lives, with the mentality of "it won't happen to me" refrain, that the problem does not get adequately addressed. Enter the financial planner who will gladly tell us how to manage our surplus, for a fee of course.

They might advise us to gamble our money away. Place the excess cash in the stock market. Yet, in this case-scenario, who makes the money? More often than not it is these money brokers who make money with their commissions and transaction fees. The regular "Joe" has to pay to play. You pay to get in and you pay to get out. If you have made some equity on your invested capital, the government is there for their "cut" of the "winnings": capital gain. By the time it is all said and done there is not much left in the personal coffers for the average hardworking American to shake a stick at. Some will say a "gain" is better than a "loss." And this, I believe, is true in most circumstances, but, with the puny amount that is left over after the bills of monthly living are paid, it is barely enough to get you an entrance fee into the eldercare institutions when, in very short order, these institutions will have spent all that money and then garner house and home.

Not to worry, these institutions have financial planning departments to help you part with all worldly possessions before it's your time for the grave. Could these factors play a role in why we see so many homeless people roaming the streets, begging for a handout, sleeping under bridges and in old abandoned houses or doorways? Walk around the District of Columbia a little, and you will see all the homeless begging for the tax-dollar handout. It is a sight, and a sore one at that! And what makes it all the more painful is that many have come to accept this as the norm. And so it is.

So humans have run into the problem of storing surpluses. People look to things that will hold up to the test of time and hold value, not to be eaten away by inflation, encouraging the free-flowing velocity of money. Money needs to flow in order for commerce to function as it does! Money is the grease that lubricates the economic wheels of a free market. This is, I like to imagine, why people like to buy gold.

It doesn't rot like, say hay, or grain in a barn. It takes up less space to store, you can confidently "bury" it to hide it and protect it from scoundrels like the banker, broker, or even taxman—or so it used to be—and it will not deteriorate, rust, or rot, from a human perspective. The funny thing about gold is: what do you do with it? Make jewelry? That's good, but it doesn't, by itself, heat the house or put food on the table. I've never witnessed someone buying groceries at the supermarket, in this day and age, paying with gold bullion or even gold coin, for that matter. I guess it could happen but probably unlikely. And yet, stranger things have happened. It is not like in the day of bartering, when you could pay the doctor with a few chickens, maybe some eggs, and a pig, and so forth. You get the picture. So what need does the farmer in Cambodia have of surplus? He has no place to store it and possibly—learning to trust no one—no interest in it either. Not being much interested in working hard for another, who, under the guise of gain, takes the proceeds for themselves. Prevalent in Western societies, where "Big-Money" moves "Big Commodities," the little one loses on many levels.

Surplus does, on the other hand, free up time. The efficiency that humans have developed in providing for the necessities of life has freed up time for adventure, exploration, and the arts, for some, like never before. People in advanced societies have more free time than ever before. Free time, as many have come to know, can be a dangerous thing. Some people are not so constructive with their free time, and there are now many more distractions to lead people astray than ever before. Vice has been around for a long, long time and only seems to advance with the "good life." Distractions from the truth abound with abandon. Religion is a form of governance. It seems like today in this country religion has almost become a bad word. Many in positions to make positive contributions to society have squandered the opportunity away to selfish endeavors—some on a very evil, demented highway to hell, squandering others hard earned surplus.

Many "innocents" have paid a high price. Many victims to greed and perversions; "Nothing new under the sun."

Surplus is a double-edged sword, which we have welded of our own making into a wild-ride without ending in sight. And yet we have the means to make corrections and redirect surplus. One of the problems is incompetence. In the halls of society incompetence abounds. And yet there is a difference between incompetence and apathy. Wouldn't it be nice if all were able to find their true vocations where apathy might abate and society would have a place for all to be competent toward more equitable distribution of surpluses. And yet, we, as a society, just seem to be slipping more and more into the abyss. It may not be too late, but then it may be. Nevertheless, it is hope that we hold onto, and with hope we venture into the unknown looking for a cure. One thing is for sure: without hope we have nothing.

TECHNOLOGICAL COSTS

The medical profession can now keep people "alive" a lot longer than nature, or God, of some sorts, if you like, seemed to intend.

Through drugs and/or artificial mechanical means, such as controlled respiration/ventilation, people are kept alive a lot longer than without this technically advanced know-how. It is remarkable what the management of breathing can do with the internal biochemistry of the human being.

I, as a Respiratory Practitioner, can manipulate the breathing of a human being such that I can increase the blood/oxygen saturation of the patient just by the mechanical manipulation of the intubated patient's breathing pattern via the ventilator (breathing machine), even without supplemental $O2$ (although acutely critically ill patients in the ICU generally, these days, almost always are placed on supplemental $O2$).

Through real-time monitoring I can watch a patient's blood-oxygen saturation climb quickly and markedly with a few turns of some buttons on the breathing-machine. I can quickly increase the purging of $CO2$ from the blood and, verifiably, via bedside blood gas analysis, note marked changes in the potential of hydrogen (pH) of the blood and hence throughout the body in a life-sustaining systems-wide flow. At times it seems almost sacrilegious, going against the wishes of God. This is, of course, if you are a God-fearing person. Otherwise, it is just another day in the "live" laboratory called—in the medical profession—the ICU.

Doctors, so it seems, are taught to put such notions of a God aside and have no particular bent toward a higher power in their thoughts and actions.

Technology is the higher power for many. Doctors believe THEY are the higher power. All must bend to them. This may be why doctors find themselves in an awkward position when faced with the imminent death of a patient. But, who's to say: have we not seen the patient who's lost all hope; medical care withdrawn: removal of the ventilator and breathing tube, stopping breathing assistance of any kind altogether; no more life-supporting drugs; comfort measures only (CMO); some narcotics and maybe some supplemental O2 (for some reason—I think it makes the doctors and nurses feel better because they are "doing something").

Then, with the patient extubated, the first words out of their mouth: "I'm starving! Can I get a turkey sandwich please?" They are moved out of the ICU to the medical ward, then after a time off to rehab and then home to live another day. The doctor has a hard time explaining that one but, notwithstanding, takes the credit for saving a life. Oh the ironies of life, and death.

These families say medicine works in the hands of God (some do say this). Maybe. But this kind of thing does not happen very often; enough though for many to hold out hopeless hope, and again: without hope we have nothing.

Not all avenues of life-sustaining technology are utilized all the time. Cost is, and has been, in one way or another, a big factor. As from time immemorial, caring has always costs time and resources, as has been discussed. Unlike some modalities and drugs, like supplemental O2, which, in some facilities, gets handed out like candy at Christmas time, not all technology is approved for all cases. It is wise to remember: too much of a good thing can be detrimental to your health and wellbeing—your life. Oxygen is one of those things.

Most doctors seem to be clueless as to the adverse effects free oxygen radicals circulating with an electron imbalance—ROS—have within the body of a living being. The doctors fresh out of school anyway appear to fail to make the connection; nevertheless, the free radicals, often times, do not; they, the ROS's, make the connection to the detriment of the host. An old term is oxygen toxicity. Yes, it is true: oxygen in high doses is toxic. Like the song says: "love is like oxygen. You get too much you get too high, not enough and your gonna' die."

Oxygen is so toxic some believe that if the Food and Drug Administration (FDA) had been born before the revelation of the oxygen molecule, and the havoc it can wreak with life, it never would have been approved as a medical gas. These free radicals can wreak havoc in the chemistry of life itself. Another one of the ironies of life I suppose. Like the effects of the sun; life would not exist as we know it without sunlight, and yet it is sunlight that can destroy the structures that sustain life itself, just like the O_2 molecule. Where would we be without trees?

Advanced medicine is incredible—truly, indeed, incredible. The knowledge and understanding of the functions of the human body and life's processes are truly astounding. The lives that have been saved and the quality of life that has been improved due to medical knowhow is truly amazing, to say the least. The technology adapted to this knowledge is no less impressive. Unless, of course, insurance is not going to reimburse, then some modalities and the impressiveness become moot, no doubt, being eliminated as an option by the third-party payer. Take for example ECMO technology and its potential role in the rapid onset of acute ARDS, where the lungs are compromised, for vast and varied reasons, such as a blunt-force trauma to the chest, as in an automobile accident, or sepsis. The lung parenchyma becomes compromised in a very complex and, still yet to be completely understood, damaging way. Sometimes reversible, many times not. The mortality rate for ARDS patients is high. ECMO has the potential to change this.

Oxygen and other critical gasses, like carbon dioxide, stop moving from lung to blood and blood to lung in ARDS. It is very difficult to get oxygen to the blood and ultimately to the vital organs in a diseased or damaged (or both) lung. So death eventually ensues in many, many, cases. ECMO can bypass the lungs and put oxygen directly into the blood and remove the CO_2, like they do during open-heart 'bypass' surgeries in the surgical suite. This technology, hypothetically, in ARDS cases can keep the patient alive while the lungs have time to heal. But it is a very expensive technology. The equipment is intricately sensitive and expensive, and technicians to operate this equipment are expensive, and hard to come by too. There are many compromised cardiac patients here today in the U.S. thanks to corporate America enabling poor lifestyles. Heart surgeries today pays the institutions and surgeons very well so no ECMO for ARDS patients; too expensive.

On other technological fronts it is a dangerous and difficult operation to transport critically ill patients to these technically advanced diagnostic testing labs, such as to the CT scanner or MRI suite, which are usually at a distance from the ICU's. These critically ill patients are in no mood or condition to be moved around or even touched; many do not like even being turned in the bed. My point is: critically ill patients do not like to be moved as I've said. Therefore to take a patient who has many life-lines (intravenous and arterial) attached—catheters, artificial airways, and tubes— of which are at risk of being erroneously crimped or displaced by accident can be life-threatening. As mentioned, these patients have no reserve to fall back on. Most all of these patients' vital organs are dependent on artificial technological means to keep the system whole and alive. Traveling through the hallways of a large institution creates challenges in the act itself, even when one is healthy and mobile. Now throw in beds, equipment, and refuge strewn about the hallways, visitors and other patients moving about, or waiting for an elevator—all lend themselves to impending disaster.

Here is an example: on one particular night a nurse, nurse's aide, and respiratory therapist are traveling back from the CT scanner with an intubated critically ill patient being ventilated with a "transport" ventilator, which is being manned and pushed alongside the patient's bed. This ventilator must be kept within close proximity to the patient to prevent a life-threatening extubation from an inadvertent pull on the vent circuit if moved too far from the bed.

Heading back to the ICU with the patient in a new technologically advanced "autonomous" bed, which is supposed to drive itself, trouble ensues. The bed has hand controls at the head for the nurse to aide in steering, if necessary. The technology for this institution is new, and the nurse "driving" this particular night is not well versed in its operation. She should not have even been driving. But she was.

[Some nurses think they are infallible. These are the most dangerous nurses. Incompetent nurses living on others' past reputations, when nurses could do no wrong, have lead many astray. Boy how times have change behind the curtain.]

This poorly driving nurse is continuously bouncing the bed off the walls and doors as they proceed down the hallways and through doorways, most of which are not much wider than the beds themselves. Going through one of these very narrow doorways the bed slams into the metal emergency panic/crash bar on the door and tears apart the chest-tube tube that is hanging over the side of the bed going from the patient's chest to the vacuum-pack hanging on the lower-level hooks at the foot of the bed. Immediately heard is a sucking sound making known instinctively the lung begins to deflate; the patient's oxygen level drops precipitously and blood pressure skyrockets along with heart rate. Critical just became deadly. The nurse says: "oops."

Here they are in the middle of the hallway, in the middle of the night, without means of communication to call for help. Quickly they proceed to the elevator—waiting, waiting, waiting—then to a harried/running push back to the ICU to where the issue could be adequately addressed and rectified. The quick-thinking respiratory therapist, while still in the hallway, tied off the torn tube stopping the pressure release of the collapsing lung, saving this patient's life.

The cost of new technology in the medical profession is mind boggling, to say the least, on many levels. One of these beds alone probably cost more than the median price of a house in this country today. And yet it really does not improve patient care all that much. The patient in the bed, I'm sure, would much rather have the money spent on sufficient and competent staff to take care of their medical needs than a bed that speaks 200 different languages. But I could be wrong.

Another example of transport intricacies (so to speak): there was this incident where a critically ill patient, being artificially ventilated, with very high concentrations of supplemental O2, maxed out on ventilatory support and cardiac medications just to keep this patient alive, finds themselves stuck in an elevator that decided not to move between floors with the doors locked shut. This went into hours before repair personnel were summoned and freed the elevator so that the patient could be brought back into the ICU. The outcome was not good.

Healthcare organizations today are all about making money toward inflating upper-managements salaries. Do they think a self-driving self-speaking bed will take the place of a well-trained nurse to save money in the long run, or are they looking to cut labor costs? The "bottom line" is all that the upper echelon seems to be concerned about. Care of the sick and infirm is just a means to that end it seems.

WE THE PEOPLE

"I was born at City Hospital in Aug. 1974. My mom says it was a hospital with a heart. They ripped up my bills when my family was denied services from the state to help pay them. My mom and dad had paid $5 a week for years at that point." Angelina Wilson, December 4, 2016: **Worcester, Mass— Places of the Past, Worcester City Hospital**

Let's take a look at the people who come to work in healthcare. In the past, as we have already noted, care of the sick and indigent was provided by the local community, which, by way of various socioeconomic reasons and maybe some "down-home" humanity, fell to the religious groups: the Church—meaning the community, for it was in these churches (not the buildings as we think of today but the people whom these buildings held), the people who make up the community would come together and decide, most democratically, so it would appear, how to conduct themselves for the greater good. They knew and felt, on many levels, God being what it is, is not always fair in the allotment of abilities distributed out to the people. Some were, and are, blessed with more abilities than others. To find one's vocation is a blessing and a beautiful thing. Many never get there. Some do find their vocation and then come to realize that the society in which they live has no need of it. But here at the beginning of communal organizations people began to realize it was not a good thing having someone die in the street. So the "good Samaritans," to use a term most fitting, took it upon themselves to educate the community to put some of their collective resources together to care for the less privileged—the sick and infirm. This, realistically, fell to the people who were blessed with unabashed compassion for humanity. These people, who had a great propensity for caring, cared for the down-and-out of their neighbors, friends, and loved ones. It didn't matter how or why these destitute came to be; the community as a whole cared about people and took charge to try to reduce the sufferings among their own.

One would be wise to remember when reading history that in days gone by people, even very well educated people at the time, did not have the hindsight we have today living in a more "advanced" age. Not letting this advanced knowledge taint our views and judgments of how and why people conducted themselves as they did in the past is of first order when studying history. Trying to put oneself in someone else's shoes, if you will, is not an easy feat (pun intended), but it is worth the effort nonetheless. Most of the people that do choose to go into a healthcare/medical profession today are money-centered persons. And what is money but a voucher to resources. These are people who pick a profession for their own living's sake. They go into medicine for the money. Many workers in healthcare today do not care about the patient; their only care is about their paychecks and the "benefits."

Here is a very interesting observation and statement I've heard said over the years which I find, through my own personal observations, to be true: "In healthcare, the further you get away from the patient the more money you make." Sad but true; in this free capitalistic society, it is not about the community or the people in it *per se*; it is all about the money. When economics calls and threatens these "not-for-profit" private healthcare organizations' income, the alarm to cut back is sounded, and who ultimately pays the price? The patients and their families, that's who.

Now, for some time, this call to "cut-back" has been resounding within the halls of the institutions we call hospitals. Every one of the direct patient caregivers has been mandated to do more with less. Well, what does that mean exactly? I'll tell you what it means: from behind the curtain, it means fewer caregivers to give care to an ever-increasing patient base and fewer supplies available to care for patients: quality has gone sub-standard; caring has gone to "crap." Management does not care. Management only cares about *their* bottom line. It is all about the money. The carrot is held out there for lower-management to decrease their budgets anyway they can, at all costs, with the possible potential perk of a big bonus to management at the fiscal year's end for a "job well done." Ouch.

In some institutions anyway, the workers are asked to cut back, "do the best you can," and do more with less. Yet, the CEO at the institution where I worked, for example, takes a 40% pay hike from one year to the next, increasing his salary from $900,000 one year to a 1.6 million dollar-a-year salary. The president of the institution took more than a 50% rise in salary, according to an article run by the Worcester Telegram some time ago. And upper and lower management can't understand why morale in the trenches is so low.

Welcome to the people in healthcare in the 21st century. The biggest complaint I hear from patients—as I've noted above—is that the people who give the care have no compassion. This should not come as any surprise in this day and age in the United States. When people are overworked and under paid and expected to do a good job without the resources to achieve that good job, it affects their outlook on life. Then add the bent of a capitalistic way of life; people get tired of working so hard to make other people rich. The bottom line is, in reality, people going into the profession of healthcare, within its many facets and disciplines today, have no interest in health care; they are all about their own concern: Money! They only care about the money! Why would a sickly person in a hospital listen to an extremely obese, unhealthy-looking healthcare provider, huffing and puffing while barging into the patient's room, stinking of cigarette smoke, listen to anything she, or he has to say about good health? Why? I am a big proponent of teaching by example, not the "do as I say, not as I do" mentality.

Unhealthy attitudes promote unhealthy actions. And this is why healthcare today is so profitable. These institutions are not about making people well. There is no money in that. These institutions are all about securing revenue for future profits and therefore go about "their" business in making more people sick. It is like going to an unscrupulous auto mechanic to get the problem with your car fixed. You go in with one problem and come out with two more. Once they've got you in the system, they are hell-bent on keeping you there. If you have health insurance, as now the law requires all to have, the hospital administration is not going to let you go until all the available cash has been excised (to use a medical term for effect) from the account. Just like many dentists in the area today. They work toward sinking their teeth into those available funds. Insurance companies play the game too and now are implementing life-limits on amounts spent in ones mouth. I have seen doctors make up diagnoses and order drugs and treatments when there is no indication to treat. It's all about billing, all about the money. They know how to play the capitalist game of "gain," and they spend a lot of resources to find ways to extract this cash from the insurance companies, and/or the State, via the patients or even directly from the patient account and/or family. This is called:

104

"accounting." These institutions hide behind "bureaucracy" so no *one* is accountable. They go after your home. Have you ever seen the lines of people outside the door of the "financial help desk" at the hospital? It extends out the door and down the hall. People are distressed and sick that their illness (or pseudo-illness, of which they are clueless due to their misplaced trust in immoral doctors, nurses, and administrators) is putting them in the poorhouse or, more accurately these days, out on the street.

Now, I've mentioned the doctors who, in order to satisfy quotas (they will tell you there are no quotas), will make a diagnosis to get the patient admitted. This is all dependent on the third-party payer. If there is money in the account to be "had," the "organization" will go after it. This sounds like fraud. And I say: IT IS!

Let me give you an example. As a Respiratory Care Practitioner I get a call about a newly admitted patient with an admitting diagnosis of COPD. As I review the medical record, this diagnosis seems out of place. There is no history of cigarette smoking; there is no family history of COPD; there is no history of Alfa-1 Antitrypsin deficiency; there is no record of a pulmonary functions test (PFT) being done on this patient. Ever! The nurse's assessment reads: "breath sounds clear; breathing unlabored; cough unproductive; vital signs good; pt. in no respiratory distress."

Upon entering the room I find a pleasant 62-year-old woman sitting up comfortably in bed, watching TV. I make sure I have the correct patient: I address her by her first name, which I have on record, and ask her last name. She tells me, and the names match up. I ask her date of birth. She answers correctly. I determine I have the correct patient for the doctor's order for respiratory breathing treatments.

[In this particular institution the protocol is for any pt. admitted with a diagnosis of COPD, the initial start of in-house "breathing" treatments will be every four hours (q4hrs) for the first 24 hours, then the respiratory therapist can "score" the pt in a standardized protocol to determine the appropriate and necessary treatment frequency based on present symptoms and history. Most physicians do not like this loss of control and will therefore write "Out of Protocol", meaning the treatments will be given q4hrs (whether the treatments are needed or not) until the doctor writes a specific order to discontinue (d/c) such treatments.]

Now this particular 62-year-old female patient, as I come to find out through my conversation with her, came to the hospital via ambulance due to a fall, resulting in an ankle injury.

"How is your breathing?" I ask.

"Fine" she replies.

I listen to her breath sounds—auscultation with a stethoscope—breath sounds clear. I ask her if she has ever taken a breathing treatment before or ever had any breathing medicine.

"No, never! Except for today on the ambulance ride over here." She continues, "I don't know why they gave that to me?"

[Please note: this institution operates much of the EMS ambulance services within this city and its surrounding towns]

I continue my assessment, asking: "Have you ever had a pulmonary functions test, where they have you blow into a machine, or sit in a booth and measure your breathing?"

"No!"

"Have you ever heard of 'COPD' associated with your health?"

"No, never!"

"Okay. Well the doctor has ordered you for breathing treatments every four hours."

"Why?"

Good question!

COPD is the admitting diagnosis. And so this scenario plays out time and time again. When the issue of fraud is brought up to the respiratory director and supervisors, therapists are told: "Just give the neb."

Heading to TBM?

I have seen many a doctor order many a breathing treatment for very small children just to pacify the parents so as to be able to say, "we treated," ('and now have something billable') "you can go home now." I have seen many a doctor order rescue breathing medication for children to have one treatment "for the road," as they like to say, discharging the patient. Really! Give a rescue emergency medication and then send them out the door. Children? What kind of medicine are they "practicing?" Do we not "practice" evidence-based medicine? Where is the evidence showing this type of treatment being good for these types of patients? Manipulated medicine—that's where you will find it—in the fabricated studies of numbers coming out of these institutions. Why do you think pediatric asthma is on the rise in this country? I'll tell you why: because doctors make it a diagnosis—so that the third party will pay—every time some parent brings their child to the ER with a runny nose. So, many times the doctor hears wheezing sounds and orders a bronchodilator because they assume the patient is in bronchospasm? Bedside PFT's are not beyond reach, they just need funding. I have resolved many a wheeze by having the patient take a deep breath, hold it for a count of 10, and then a strong cough on the way out. Secretions can act like a "reed" in the airway, and be very "musical." Once the secretions are cleared by the best method out there, a cough, the wheezing quickly, and to many's, even the doctor's, amazement, and is miraculously gone. No drugs yet great pulmonary therapy. Of course this is more difficult in the very young, and, in the infant, nature plays the role for the most part: involuntarily. They do not have asthma; they are suffering from a bout of the common cold. But the third-party does not pay for that. Insurance does not cover a cough or the common cold, as far as I know.

ER rooms and staff are expensive, no doubt. Just like in a restaurant, you cannot sit at a table and not pay. The institution has no interest in letting someone occupy a room, drink juice and soda, have a turkey sandwich, and not bill for it. This is revenue-based medicine. If a child is in such respiratory distress that they need to be given a rescue medication, should they really be walking out the hospital door at three in the morning? We all know the logical and responsible answer to this question: "NO, they should not!" So what is really going on here? The doctor surely cannot be stupid. Doctors have many years of schooling and have the paper that says it is so. So now the question really is: does the doctor really know best? Most people do not like my answer to that question. Is ignorance really bliss? I'll leave it to you, the reader, to decide for yourself.

HYPOCRATIC STAFF

I'll repeat: I'm a big proponent of "teach-by-example"—I may not always be good at it, but I make a conscious effort—and find it strange that a respiratory therapist would come in from just smoking a cigarette—stinking of smoke—and go give a breathing treatment to a patient suffering from a pulmonary disease. My thought, being in such a profession: the "professional" should be promoting good pulmonary hygiene by example. Why would someone listen to someone else go on and on about the need for healthy behavioral modifications when coming from a person who is really only thinking about when they can step outside and have another "smoke break" and how long till the next payday? I've heard new recruits in orientation say "I like orienting with smokers because we go on break more often." Counterproductive? Yes, and on so many levels—to say the least—it is hypocritical. Not to mention (but of course I will) knowing full well the gruesome details of a death from lung disease and all the objective evidence out there as to the ravishing effects of the disease, and cancers, attributed directly to the exposure of tobacco products. I have a hard time fathoming that these people in the profession, with specific education on the intricacies of pulmonary functions, health, and diseases of the lungs, would do such a thing as smoke cigarettes. Addictions are strong; I understand this. The only thing I can come up with is: they feel, "if I only have a few good years left, I'm going to enjoy them. And I enjoy smoking cigarettes." Ok then.

Still, these "professional" people, who know the sufferings ahead and continue in that direction, continue to baffle me. Lung disease is just that: "without ease." It is true: "When you can't breathe, nothing else matters." It is a slow, painful, miserable death. Most all-available energy, O2, is used up just in the feeble attempt to breathe with lung disease. But, like some say, "life is short; you never know when your time is up!" And, I'd have to agree. Nevertheless, it just might be, that there will be a "tomorrow." Some say it is wise to have somewhat of a tentative plan to face the morrow, and what it may bring.

Finding a balance is not always easy, but why stack the cards against yourself and drag others down with you? Do we really live in a careless, sadistic world?

Things in this society change, as all things do, and, in this society, sometimes when they change, they change fast. I remember when banning cigarette smoking from all public buildings here in Massachusetts first went into effect. Now it is just a fact of life. But really it was not that long ago when they first tried "smoking" and "non-smoking" areas in public places. That was a joke. I remember taking a bus trip from California to New Hampshire back in the late 70s: a five-day, and night, trip from California to New Hampshire. The back of the bus was the smoking area. Lots of people smoked then in the 70s; the whole bus was just full of smoke. It didn't matter if you went all the way up to the front of the bus—the "no smoking area"—the whole bus was a cloud of smoke; the bus driver would usually be smoking too. But those were different times, and information about the deleterious effects of smoking tobacco was just beginning to come to the forefront.

I like to tell the story of years ago when going into the hospital, say, as a visitor, and you walk around the corner and come in view of the nurses' station: nurses sitting around this "off-to-the-side" table, or maybe even a round table in the middle, behind the work counter, where the patient charts were kept, smoking cigarettes. The ashtray overflowing with cigarette butts and light gray cigarette ashes with a matching cigarette-smoke plume billowing in the air that seemed to just hover above and then sweeps into a swirling dancing motion as one or two nurses come and go from tasks of answering a patient's call button, or bathroom light, or what have you. A doctor waltzes in, sits down with the nurses at the table, lights up a cigarette and starts "chatting-up" the nurses, who, by the by, at this point in American history, were predominantly female and the doctors mostly male. Oh how things have changed. Some, of course, for the better; some not so much!

> Male roles in nursing were minimal where I worked until the 90s; nursing is still a predominantly female profession; doctors not so much. It has become a women's world here in the United States of America.

Some of those call-lights the nurses would attend to would be a patient complaining about the smoke coming from the patient next to him or her. Yup, that's right, smoking in bed, in the hospital, within a hyper-oxygenated environment. Doctor knows best?

Now we may be tempted to say: "what were they thinking?" But, as we all know, in a capitalistic "free" market "money-grubbing" society, money rules. And each is "free" to choose how he or she goes about getting as much of it as they can—within reason, and the confines of the law, of course. There are some rules but, really, many more loopholes. The object is to get as much as you can and try to get more than anyone else, at any cost. As the Orient calls the Occident: "crab culture."

For some people it is not only about the money, it seems, but also, and maybe more importantly, about how one shows it. The mentality is: if no one knows just how wealthy you are, then what good is it? So many people like to flaunt. Nothing new. Probably why gold has stood the test of time. People generally like to be flashy. Gold works well on that front in the form of jewelry. And it makes sense. For a community to survive and expand, its members need to procreate, and what better way to attract a mate than with a flashy allure. Just as the angler lures them in!

And, of course, people love toys, toys of all kinds. But, best of all, toys that will impress one's neighbors and friends! So any excess, or any credit, goes into, sometimes, big and expensive toys. I call it bric-a-brac, which really is nothing more than sentimental crap. "Fools we are for our desires."

Nevertheless, as I state over and over, the "hospital" staff, top to bottom, seems all about the money in today's healthcare industry. Patient-care comes second. The administration will never say such a thing and 'trench' workers get on board or get out.

Let me give you another example of the types of people who are working in and directing healthcare today. The director of the Respiratory Care Department pushes nebulizer treatments.

This is confounding, because there are other, better modes these days for delivering respiratory medications. The only time a nebulizer treatment is necessary is when the patient is in such distress that they cannot speak in full sentences for need of taking another breath or cannot hold their breath for any period of time. When using the metered dose inhaler (MDI), the preferred way to take inhaled breathing medication (some prefer even newer, and considered better, modalities than the MDI's to deliver breathing medications like dry caplets and others), one must be able to do a breath hold and, ideally, hold the breath for a count of 10, or 10 seconds. This extends the time the medication is in the lungs and allows for absorption by the lung tissue, resulting in rapid maximal efficacy. The problem management has with MDI's is they cost a lot more than a nebulizer treatment.

SO: "Just give the neb!" Needed or not.

MOVING FORWARD
(OR BACK?)

It has been said that if you really want to test a relationship: go camping. Spending a few days roughing-it in the wilderness, people tend to show there, their "true-colors" quickly. These trips have been known to "make or break" a relationship. So with this knowledge at hand I bring to light Moses and the Israelites. Certainly these adventurers must have learned something about living together, and the intricacies of community during their 40 years of camping out in the desert. They must have come to experience a whole assortment of communal difficulties with people living in such close proximity to one another. Everyone must have had a very particular role to play for the smooth functioning of their society. All must have been integral and with import, right down to the most mundane tasks such as, oh, let's say, cleaning the latrine; dealing with shit. Certainly we know today no task can be pushed aside but to the whole's own detriment.

Sanitation becomes a huge issue, and a community learns quite quickly what is acceptable and what is life-threatening in a big way. Epidemics can very well be the end of a whole people and tend to occur when populations begin to proliferate and waste becomes a big problem. History teaches, and ancient books depict, just how a community might conduct itself to live in peace, harmony, tranquility, health, and accord. So let's take a look at the community of the Israelites of old and the hospitals of the communities today.

Community and the institution have come together through a long journey of trial and error—and still proceed into the future as such, pretty much

113

"feeling" their way through the dark. Practicing? Practice, practice, practice! The unique thing about humans is their ability to pass on information from the past. Intelligent is the one who learns from the mistakes of others. God bless those who, with great foresight, and fortitude, knew enough to start writing these things down. We owe everything to the past. Unfortunately, for the loser, history is written by the victor and biased toward the whims of the conqueror's scribes. Many have written just to keep their own heads on. Notwithstanding, one is wise to read "between-the-lines." So now, let's bring the past up into the present to see where the future might lead. And, at the same time, go back to the wanderings-in-the-wilderness, some of the lessons the community learned through all their long adventures to survive.

Moses of old seemed to have had a pretty good understanding of how power corrupts. The laws, which he descended Mount Ararat with, seem to directly address such momentous issues in striving for the healthy, longstanding direction of a community.

The Ten Commandments seem, to me, a good place to start; they seem to be well known (I could be wrong) and well documented throughout history.

The Decalogue:

[I paraphrase]

I) You shall have no other gods before me.

2) You shall not make idols.

3) You shall not take the name of the LORD your GOD in vain.

4) Remember the Sabbath day: keep it holy.

5) Honor your father and your mother.

6) You shall not murder.

7) You shall not commit adultery.

8) You shall not steal.

9) You shall not bear false witness against your neighbor.

10) You shall not covet.

The first five address the individual's and the community's relationship with God—keeping with a strong effort not to put any one in such a standing as to lead without impunity. Six thru 10 deal with the relationships within the community itself. Parents are to be revered for the very fact that procreation is a Godly act. To bring life into this world or the very fact of creating a life, of any kind, is beyond human understanding, and yet, a complex life form such as a human is, in my estimation, nothing less than miraculous: "an act of God. "Let's take a look at each one individually, shall we, and how it is viewed within the medical profession. Or not!

This is a presentation of an individual's perspective (mine) of communal life as it has come down to us through the passage of time and history and how it has, or has not, played out within the institution of hospital.

The first commandment tells us to "have no other gods before me." It seems to me that doctors, within the medical community, and in the doctors' minds themselves, more often than not, have redefined God as their own persona turned adulterated anima. God has no place in the halls of medicine it seems. One can only imagine how today if a doctor came into the OR suite and said to the staff, "Ok, now, let's all get on our knees and pray before we begin the procedure."

The second commandment of the Hebrew Bible tells us not to "make idols." So what is an idol? In the medical profession the doctor expects to be idolized. After all "they" are God, in their own minds—some of them anyway. This is very perceptive, for, if taken in context, some may bow. I also have a great amount of respect for and love of information and education, thankful for the written word and for the people who take the time to write down information so that others to come can learn and grow toward a better way of life for all. This may be a little romantic, unrealistic, and farfetched. The educational opportunity doctors have had is not to be squandered. I have a great amount of respect for the amount of education these medical doctors have. The amount of knowledge in medicine is expanding so fast; it must be next to impossible to keep up. Which is why, I think, so many medical doctors have become disciplined specialists—so refined that the problem is bringing them all together in a unified and consorted whole. Doctors sometimes have a hard time communicating with each other, so it seems. It may be surprising for some to think the medical "God," called "doctor," does not know all. Many doctors come across as if they do. One thing I've learned over the years in dealing with many, many of doctors, from great, well-seasoned, brilliant doctors to interns right out of med school – I repeat to drive the point: arrogance is just a mask ignorance hides behind. Make no mistake about it. The renowned physician is very well aware of the human limitations within himself or herself and does not try to hide the fact from the patient; they will give their word to find out as much about the case as possible, and, the big difference is: the great ones do. These are the doctors who know they are here on this earth to DO Gods work not to *be* God.

Three: "You shall not take the name of the LORD your GOD in vain." I have found myself on more than one occasion cursing the doctor on my way home from a very difficult shift in the ICU or the ER. I am human. I've heard doctors curse themselves. The real curse is in being a perfectionist here in this imperfect world.

Four: "Remember the Sabbath day, to keep it holy." This is an unknown concept in the hospital but for the devout. I remember one time I exited the locked entrance into the ICU, and outside this door, as I exited, was a doctor who wanted me to let him in—I am not supposed to let anyone in who is unknown to me and is not authorized to be in the unit. Visiting is restricted to family members only and authorized personnel, for the most part, and employees must show a badge identifying themselves, and, if they have a badge and are authorized to enter, they can 'swipe' themselves in. When I inquired further, of this very "new" young-looking doctor, as to why he didn't have his badge. He replied that he, for religious reasons, could not use any electronic devices, this being the Sabbath. I was suspicious, for he did not show me any ID, and I did not recognize him. I replied that maybe he was in the wrong profession. I would have some concern as to having this doctor participating in a emergent event on the Sabbath where someone's life is on the line and if he cannot use electronic devices like cardiac monitors or a defibrillator on the patient in cardiac arrest. Medical studies have shown this equipment, very often, to have good effect in helping save people's lives.

Five: "Honor your father and your mother." Too many times I have seen doctors keep elderly people alive way too long, disregarding their patients' wishes and "using" them as long as they can to run the patients bill up before letting them die. Death without dignity is a disgraceful and a disturbing thing to witness. I've witnessed it all too often. I propose legislation be passed requiring any patient, let's say, over the age of 70, who enters the ER or, for that matter, any medical facility, seeking any kind of medical treatment, has Hospice involved – I talk further on this below -- in educating, not only the patient, but the whole family as well, near and far, on what is to come. Hospice from an outside source must be required, for if in-house palliative care is implemented, the institution is apt to sway things to their own bottom-line. That is, they are apt to focus on money instead of education in the realities of death and all its vast and varied ramifications for those who are coming to the close of their years on this earth and also the family in letting go. After all life IS one big lesson in letting go. And from what I've seen, even those who think they are prepared for the death of a loved one, never really are. The emotions run high and wild, of which many, unless they have been through it before, can never imagine. It is not an easy thing for all involved. Don't let anyone fool you. Education is the key to easing the difficult moment of death. Saying your last goodbyes is very surreal. Hospice has the knowledge and the tools. Require them to share it. They are an incredible resource, which, I believe, is underutilized, and, because of this, people suffer more than may be necessary.

Six: "You shall not murder." Murder? Is negligence considered murder? Is incompetence considered murder? Semantics?

I'm not sure of the legal ramifications for such ineptitude, but what really bothers me is the matter-of-fact attitude, such as "just another day at the office" by many medical "professionals." Complacent disregard for human decency, to me, is a form of unmitigated murder. If a lack of human compassion is the order-of-the-day, and someone dies because of it, what is that? There must be accountability. Murder is a very strong word, and it makes me cringe when I see healthcare professionals lose compassion or, even worse, never even considered it. Very unprofessional to say the least! Management makes it easy for themselves by avoiding the dirty truth of the trenches. Incompetence abounds.

Seven: "You shall not commit adultery." Adultery? There are many improprieties that take place behind the curtain, or closed doors, if you like, in these large institutions we call hospitals. Take for instance the two lesbian nurses (I don't know if they were married, such marriages in Massachusetts, at the time, were lawful), who thought, I suppose, it would be fun to seduce a male doctor (I didn't know if he was married, either), who willingly decides, during working hours, when patient care is the reason for their being there, to engage in a "threesome" sexual escapade in a backroom. These three's improprieties were only revealed because they were being "loud," and someone overheard the noise coming from behind closed doors and "blew the whistle" (to use a phrase). Now I'm not weighing in on the rightness or wrongness of such sexual bents, but if you're going to do it, do it on your own time. I see shunning responsibilities to patient care for personal gratification, while employed to care for patients, as adulterous. But that's just me.

Eight: "You shall not steal." These institutions are stealing the community blind. Overbilling; unnecessary procedures; unnecessary testing; unnecessarily medicating: unethical activities such as intubating the unruly patient because they keep screaming to be discharged? What to do, what to do? These are not easy situations, to say the least, but where is patient dignity in intubating to shut them up? Well, there is no dignity in that, but there is a lot of revenue to be had. You must remember the doctor is given God-like status and expects never to be questioned. The doctor "always knows best," and I write this with tongue in cheek over and over again. The doctor does not always know best. Sometimes doctors can be your worst enemy in today's healthcare market. Now you're in the healthcare "system," and at the very mercy of this system, for the quagmire gets very murky very fast behind the curtain. You may have heard the term "falling through the cracks," but this is being way too kind to the medical community that only seems to care about the money.

Nine: "You shall not bear false witness against your neighbor." I believe fraud is rampant in the medical profession these days. People steal from the institution for their own personal gain, large and small alike. Is it not stealing when, just before allowing a terminally ill patient to 'pass' the doctor orders and sends the patient to a barrage of testing? For what, why another CT scan and an MRI before signing a CMO order and *then* withdrawing care? Why, to generate revenue?

As I've stated these diagnostic equipment like CT scanners are very expensive to purchase and maintain; these and other testing equipment the institution does not like to go idle. Being idle does not pay the bills. Why would a family member allow a doctor to put a loved one through more suffering and distress before they are allowed to die? Yes, the medical profession, in today's technologically driven society, makes these decisions as to when one stops breathing. I have seen more cruel and abusive treatment by medical professionals of their charges than I'd like to remember. This is how I've come to refer to the ICU as a torture chamber.

And Ten: "You shall not covet." "Covet"; the Merriam-Webster dictionary states its number two meaning as a transitive verb: "to desire inordinately or culpably." This last commandment seems to reflect and sum up all the others before it, and the first seems to encompass the whole. Which, in and of itself can be beautiful in its simplicity, and yet so difficult to understand, never mind putting into practice. So for me, and I'm confident I'm not alone; God is the ultimate absolute being of profound love, way beyond human understanding or comprehension. Although, working in the ICU, many times I have said to myself, on my ride home after working a tough case: "where is the God in that!?"

So these commandments try to give direction and helpful advice to a community along the way. The last is the epitome of evil: Pride. To covet is to move away from community, becoming so self-absorbed and myopic as to see the world we find ourselves in, and our perception of it, absolute. The ancient book of wisdom the "Tao" teaches that flexibility is the key to life, while rigidity leads to death. One bends when stressed while the other snaps and breaks.

SOCIAL COST

Over a span of about five years, maybe more, at least five well-seasoned and respected therapists within the discipline of Respiratory Care have come to be expelled from the institution of which I write, for various reasons, some legitimate, I suppose, some questionable. These particular colleagues and friends came to their demise by various means within a year or two upon leaving employment of this hospital. Dead early! Some from suspicious causes maybe, never officially disclosed; some for reasons never discovered; another simply went into the basement and put a rope around his neck. Nevertheless, all dead within a year or two after being terminated by the "institution."

On a microcosmic scale we can see the cost paid by the players, unwittingly or not. The change comes where health care institutions are run as a business—I don't care if you want to call it "for-profit" or "not-for-profit"—where business people are concerned: the "bottom line" is all that seems to matter. The revenue gets accounted for in nice, neat—even if in sometimes obscure and deceitful ways—columns of debits and credits. The larger the institution, the longer the columns and therefore the numbers; when dealing in percentages it must become easier to overlook the "nuances of the patients" (and employees) in this particular scenario. I see healthcare executives not caring at all about patient care, or about their employees' care, either—only about the bottom line. I believe "healthcare" is supposed to be a community service, serving the communities health and wellbeing—the commonweal—ultimately creating a very healthy and vibrant community "whole." My point, in the broad sense, is that not only the community members at large, who seek medical care, deserve to be treated with dignity and respect and receive the best medical care available, but also the health care givers themselves. These institutions need to be honestly and truly promoting healthy habits of all types for all peoples, as in: work, leisure, study, and/or play for everyone. I don't see this being the case today. The business people at the helm seem only to be looking at the bottom-line and tacking to meet good results from a business standpoint.

Now I must interject here that I am acutely aware of the importance of the bottom line. Accounting practices and balanced-sheets do not elude me completely. I am aware that bills need to be paid.

To continue: I will give you some examples of what becomes of some professionals for reasons one can only deduce from apparent facts, which, by the way, usually are not facts at all, but secondhand gossip. So I'll present the scenario as close to facts as possible, being brief, and leave any drawing of conclusions to the subjective nature of you the reader.

HIPAA

(Health Insurance Portability and Accountability Act)

In this day and age, with the tight federal regulations about personal medical records, hospital medical employees—the people who work with and around patients and their medical records—upon learning that a co-worker becomes ill or is out of work sick for an extended period of time (more than 4 days), are seemingly timid or afraid to ask too many questions for fear of a HIPAA violation. So many, as a result, will not ask at all. This could give the ill co-worker a feeling of isolation and even rejection in a way: making them feel even more ill, possibly. On the other hand some can be, shall we say (to be polite) completely uncaring.

PETE

One day my old high school classmate, friend, and longtime colleague, Pete, just stopped coming to work. Just stopped!

Now, just around Christmas time before he stopped coming to work, Pete comes in to work his scheduled nightshift and finds his locker door closed. Locked. Now Pete never locked or even closed his locker door due to the fact that the report room, where his locker was, is itself a locked room with only authorized personnel having access (respiratory therapists). So I guess some of his day colleagues thought it would be funny, after so many years, to have Pete come to work this Christmas eve night and find his locker door closed and locked.

The only problem they may have overlooked (maybe not) was that Pete had the combination to his locker written on a piece of white medical-tape taped to the inside of his locker. He had not committed the combination to memory. He was not happy coming to work finding his locker locked with his necessities to do his job inaccessible. I was working that night, and I found out about it from Pete not long after the shift began. Pete kept his stethoscope, his lab coat, and whatever other appurtenances he may have liked to carry while on his patient rounds in the locker. He was upset. A lot! I tried to direct him in not giving the pranksters any satisfaction by a display of anger of any kind. But he was insistent, and incensed, and posted a note upon his locker for all to see. I don't really remember what it said, something about his disgust at the "childishness" of his colleagues' actions. I felt it played right into the gag and a waste of time and energy. I was pretty sure there was a lot more behind the picture than I knew, and I thought it best to just let it go. Easy for me to say! Nevertheless, at some point not long after this incident, he stopped coming to work. I called his cell phone and was directly diverted to automated answering. This went on for a while. No one, that I remember, was talking about it but for the question: "anyone heard anything about Pete?" "No," was always the reply.

Just after a month or so Pete finally does return my phone calls and tells me he had checked into rehab for a month and that "they take everything upon admittance, cell phone; keys; credit cards; money—everything."

Pete and I would play golf together, go motorcycle riding together. We played football together in high school. Went to parties. Everyone would drink. And yes, teenagers! Eighteen was the legal "drinking" age at that time, and the group I was in was all on the older side. Many would drink to excess no doubt. But I digress.

After high school Pete and I interned at the same hospital and we both took jobs there upon completion. We worked together there for a while then went our separate ways—as life has its way of intervening—then reuniting as professional Respiratory Care Practitioners (RCP) some years later.

So I check in on Pete at his place after I find out he was home and not coming back to work anytime soon. He stopped answering his phone or returning calls at that point. I went over and, with some persistence, I suppose, got him to open the door. There were some yellow-faded-looking newspapers strewn about the door stoop as I entered. He looked a little disheveled and disoriented and discouraged. I had no idea as to what really set him in this direction. Some may say a "downward spiral," but who is really to say what works for one and not another. He told me when he was getting up in the morning his extremities would tremble uncontrollably; the only thing that would stop them was a drink of alcohol. Pete liked to drink vodka. He told me he was tired of waking up in the morning passed out on the floor. I tried to get him out of the house. I told him I wasn't there to judge, just to get him out of the house some. He told me he was being picked up a little later by his brother to go to an AA meeting. I found out later that that was a lie. He seemed, at the time, like a skittish little cat, afraid that someone was trying to snatch and cage him. I didn't push. He was trying to give me things like his furniture. He told me he was heading back to Florida. He was trying to convince me to buy his condo. I partly believed him. I did notice, as he sat in his glider by the fireplace, that there was a can of lighter fluid on the mantel with some stick matches. A quick thought flashed before me of him torching the place. Only a flash (no pun intended), and then I suppose I dismissed the thought. As my little boy and I left I told Pete I'd stop back next week to check-in on him. I got a call that week from Pete's niece.

"Pete's dead!"

"What?"

"Pete's dead! He hung himself! The neighbor saw a light on in the basement for a few days and looked in and saw Pete."

"God damn it!"

Pete chose his ending. It was not pretty; put a rope around his neck, sat down in a chair and drank himself to oblivion. There are messier ways to go. I don't blame Pete. Social costs. The job as health care provider takes its toll. Pete was 54 when he checked out.

EARL

Then there is Earl, the Respiratory Care Department's supervisor for quite a number of years. Earl had worked at this hospital for a very long time. Respiratory was his life; the institution was his life: it was his identity. And the hospital was his home. "A big Black man" as he would say, and he took pride in the fact that he was a black man who made something of himself: served his country in the military; paid his taxes; met his obligations responsibly; raised his daughter by himself; knew his respiratory therapy well; taught respiratory care at a local college at times. I do not know what exactly transpired, but when a new young respiratory female graduate, with ambitions of pushing people around and designs of becoming a supervisor—as I came to see it, she did not like people around who knew their respiratory therapy better than her—appeared to have viewed Earl as a threat, possibly due to his great breadth of knowledge in respiratory care along with the great respect and regard held for him by his many loved ones, colleagues, administrators, and patients alike. Somehow he was removed from the employs of the institution, and I don't think it was pretty. People would ask: "anyone heard about Earl?"

"No," would again be the only reply.

Earl, I had heard, had had some altercation on the outside sometime not long after being callously terminated by the institution that had benefited from his employ for so many years. At some point he ended up in the very hospital emergency room where he had worked all those years, after taking a blow to the head from a supposed roommate. I didn't really get the story, but it seems he ended up with a head bleed, intubated, ventilated in the Trauma Unit for a short stay, and then transferred to a VA hospital (being a war veteran). And then was dead in two weeks. What happened there? Earl died at 51.

SHERYL

Then we have Respiratory Therapist Sheryl, who was run out of the hospital for reasons unknown to me. Management liked to keep things hushed up and to themselves, and if anyone showed some semblance of concern, they were told: "it is not of your concern." If one presses for information they are scheduled for a visit with human resources (HR) and threatened with dismissal themselves: "The bully rule" I call it. The bully always seems to rule.

Sheryl and I had worked together for many years. We lived close by: the next town over, out in the country. I knew her Cuban husband, who was, at some point, for some reason, deported back to Cuba, so the story goes. I got to know her three children. Two were very young when their dad was taken away. I used to go over and help them out with the house. I had seen her at a medical educational seminar at one point, after she too had been thanklessly pushed out of the employs of this institution by the new wave of unscrupulous business management people making their way into the institution looking for the 'top'. Shortly after our brief reunion, I heard she was emergently admitted to another Massachusetts hospital where she died a short time later. Some said it was an asthma attack. A respiratory therapist dying of an asthma attack? I suppose it does happen. Sheryl was 43.

TERRY

Terrance, a very enthusiastic Respiratory Practitioner who loved to teach and pass on all the experience and knowledge he had gained over the years to all who had an interest: students, nurses, and doctors alike. Terry loved to teach. Terry and I became friends because that was the type of guy he was: friends with everyone. I'm not the friendly type, but Terry didn't allow that from stopping a friendship to grow between us. Terry ran into trouble with painkillers, like a lot of people in this culture today for vast and varied reasons beyond our scope here. Terry was a go-getter though, and when the drugs became a problem for him, like getting up in the morning and going to work, he took the bull-by-the-horns and went into employer-sanctioned rehabilitation. He came out with some great stories as well as a bunch of new friends, whom he would go on to help them improve their lives by his overpowering positive attitude: "never-say-can't" and many would often hear him saying "when one door closes another one opens." He jumped through all the "hoops" this hospital employer required and got his job back. He was on probation for one year and sailed through that like a true mariner. Then for some reason, again unbeknownst to me, the new wave management supervisor – the one with grand ambitions – went up to Terry one morning and asked him to pee in a cup. He refused out of principle and walked out, never to return. He was dead within a year of being cut out of this healthcare institution. "They" say: "We take care of our own." But really they do not. Terry was 59 when he passed. Still young by today's standards here in the United States where retirement from employment is more now around the age of 67 from a governments standpoint, depending on the year you were born.

JOSHUA

Josh, another colleague friend of mine, originally from Ghana, Africa, came to the U.S. and educated himself to a high level, as I came to understand. Educated at Northeastern University in science. I do not know all the specifics. Josh was a very private person and did not talk much about himself. He did however like to talk a lot about his family: his wife and two children. Josh went into respiratory therapy, he told me, because the scientific research program he was working in lost funding and closed up, so a respiratory profession was in reach and he needed to work to stay in the country.

We worked together for a very long time. Josh had had an open-heart procedure done at a Massachusetts hospital other than the one we worked at for personal and private reasons I supposed. He recovered well and returned to work when the doctors gave him the green light. As I said, Josh was a very smart man; one night some time after his heart surgery, he asks me if I could show him how to "copy-and-paste" on the computer. With Josh being from a third-world country and growing up before the computer age, I figured navigating around a computer might not be his forte. So I would show him. No big deal. We all learn at some point. But he kept asking from week to week, the same thing, over and over again. I even wrote the simple steps down for him to follow. When I was with him he seemed to do just fine, but then he would "forget." I got to the point of wondering to myself: "is he just messing with me?"

At some point the nurses in the Cardiac Unit—the unit where Josh was a "Point" therapist, meaning this was the unit where he spent most of his working hours—started complaining about "bizarre" behavioral changes in Josh's work, saying: "he's going to hurt someone." He was removed from working in the ICU and relegated to "floor-therapy-only", by management, shortly thereafter. Then he started having a hard time remembering his password to the Pyxis (locked medication dispensary cabinets) and other computer applications. Not long after this he was relieved of his duties and pressured into resigning his position at the hospital. He died within a year or two after this. It was never disclosed the cause of death but I suspected Creutzfeld/Jakob (Mad Cow) Disease. Studies have shown improperly sterilized surgical equipment can transfer the infectious agent. Josh was 64 when he died.

All died very young, by our standards, of various causes, from a "family" of respiratory therapists that, relatively speaking, is not very large. What is going on here? The job takes its toll. When working with severe suffering, death, and dying all the time, life begins to take on another meaning in some very strange ways. Respiratory therapists are always at the head of the bed of the worst of the worst cases. And they are never pretty. A child dying is a tough one. Drownings, for me are the worst. People suffering from no fault of their own takes a toll on the ones caring for them! Burnout is high among many, and yet many keep on going. Bills need to be paid. Unfortunately, the many good souls are being pushed out of the hospital, and the "money-grubbers" are swooping in.

Compassion has gone out the window in the institution. Bureaucracy and corporations make it easy for the individual to hide and shun responsibility. No ONE is responsible for the fault. How convenient! This is the world we live in today: no one takes responsibility; it is: point the finger at someone else, who, invariably, points the finger at someone else and, down the line it goes; the old adage: "shit" flows downhill. Until it gets to the one who really is not responsible, and they get all the blame, passed the buck so to speak, and not in a good way. Literally, in many directions and convoluted ways: hiding behind bureaucracy.

The "machine" is now primed. The stage has been set; the actors in place, the wheels in motion and everyone with bills to pay. One must stay actively employed to pay the rent/mortgage and taxes, which consumes a lot of time when wages—not coincidentally—are at a point, for many, where there is very little left over to spend frivolously, so to speak. And when there is some disposable income available for adventure, it, many times, leads to trouble. One does not have to look very far to see where many Americans spend disposable income, or not so easily disposed of income: tobacco, drugs and/or alcohol, and any number of unimaginable vices. It is with great irony that many a nurse and therapist, working in the ICU "torture chamber" has said, on many more than one occasion: "I can't wait for this shift to be over and have a drink!"—all the while, while on duty, caring for "train-wrecks" of patients who are suffering the adverse effects of drinking too much alcohol, or the consumption of other substances, be they licit or otherwise, or, for that matter, all the "shit" capitalist shove down our throats by way of high-powered marketing, convincing us that we just cannot live without such things.

So the job itself creates a steady patient base for future revenues. Is this by design, one might question? Conspiracy theorists would probably give a resounding: YES! Either way, eventually society always pays the cost.

Of course the business of healthcare and hospitals is a difficult one, and many, if not most, people would rather be anywhere else than in the hospital. When faced with an illness most would rather go without, without the illness that is. So subjectively speaking, it is hard to give a good review when the view can be dark and gloomy. Yet some do. Some endings are good endings, and real people give testimonies of real-life happenings with a positive experience in the long run and do not mind spreading the news. Yet in the ICU most patients are given "amnesia" type meds specifically so as to not remember much, if anything at all, of the experience. This is not a bad thing when treated responsibly, for the ICU can be a very scary place.

For instance: up in the front part of the torture-chamber unit one particular night there is this female patient in about her 60s who is going through delirium tremens (DT's): alcohol withdrawal.

[It is amazing how alcohol deteriorates the body much more quickly than if not a factor; many medical staff in the medical units will often be heard commenting on how some patients look so much older than they really are. Drug and alcohol abuse take their toll.]

Alcohol does strange things to the body, mind, and soul. This female patient was screaming at the top of her lungs the most heinous of obscenities anyone could ever have possibly heard in their entire lives. The kinds of things most people shield their children from. Very sexual in nature, like "I want to fuck you, you fucking cock sucking asshole. Fuck me, fuck me, fuck me, you fuck. Fucken' Shit, fuck me! Fuck me ..." No need for me to go on, but she did for days. And nights.

Down the back hall at this time there was a young patient in their teens who was dying—I was not involved in this case. Many young friends of the patient were coming and going to say their last goodbyes. Surreal for anyone to say a last goodbye, for these young people, it was an eye-opener to the world they were preparing to enter.

These poor young naive "adults" come walking into the unit and **BAAM**, at the top of the decibel scale: "Fuck me! Fuck me! Fuck me!" The look of fear, sorrow, worry, and disbelief on their faces in such a surreal moment was disconcerting to us all. No one could get this lady to quiet down. In many situations patients will get sedated to contain such outbursts if they are being unruly and a danger to themselves and/or the staff. This lady was a danger to herself—hence her being in four-point restraints (arms and legs tied to the bedrails)—and a danger to the staff. In the units I do not ever remember intubating to keep someone quiet; that seemed to be reserved for the ER. This particular patient screaming from the DTs was not a candidate for any heavy sedation, it was withdrawal from heavy self-medicating that the medical team was trying to get her safely through. Otherwise she could drink herself to death. And maybe that is what she was after; but loved ones very often times intervene with other ideas. It is not unusual in this ICU setting for such chaos to abound. Many times from many rooms at once. These kids were in shock by the time they walked out of the ICU. I have no doubt they had to grapple with post-traumatic stress after this harrowing experience of seeing their friend die.

JACHO JOKE

The Joint Commission on Accreditation of Healthcare (JACHO) is a joke amongst the workers within the halls of a hospitalized institution.

The history of the commission is a noble one, just as with the beginnings of the clinic and hospital: taking care of people throughout the community in deed in need. And yet, like most institutions of today, it finds itself caught-up in the vicious cycle of mammon generation from misery. The hospitals, I'm led to believe, pay handsome fees to the Joint Commission for the inspection. Getting a good score on how well the hospital is providing for the health and wellbeing of the sick and infirm of a community is of top priority. Unfortunately, the endeavor may have become perverted. Some people say everyone has their price. Meaning with enough money anyone can be bought to do just about anything. There have been a few throughout the course of history who have not succumbed, I suppose, and maybe even some today, but they usually lay low and keep their head down for fear of violent retributions.

At its inception, and for a while, JACHO gave no preannouncements to a facility of time or place of an inspection, presuming that to be a more accurate way of getting a true picture as to what goes on within the walls of the institute's 'hallowed' halls. After some complained, changes were made to announce inspection visits well in advance. A well-orchestrated itinerary of when and which units or areas of the institution JACHO inspectors were, and are, to inspect was now in hospital management's hands, allowing the institution to prepare for the upcoming inspection.

This is the joke. The Commission inspects every three years on average. This allows the hospitals administrators and management to have time to make changes on suggestions made from the last visit toward improvements in the facility. This all sounds well and good but for the fact that the hospitals are run these days by scoundrels.

The institution with which I am most familiar has the audacity to coach the "players"/employees as to what to say when the inspectors come through and to which areas at what times on which days the inspections will be conducted. It is now all prearranged as to who will be engaged in conversations, or question and answer interactions, all stealthily arranged to appear impromptu. It is one of the strangest mysteries of the world how all the extra beds, which usually line the hallways, nooks, and crannies of the hospital—clearly a fire and safety hazard—mysteriously disappear when the inspectors are coming through and then, just as mysteriously, and as quickly, reappear, from seemingly out of thin air. It is one of the most efficient systems within the hospital's operations. This system of deceit is more efficient and fine-tuned than any other, in my view, within the healthcare industry, even surpassing the art of medicine itself. This system of hiding "failings" and "shortcomings" is truly amazing. Instead of working to sincerely correct any shortcomings, the hospital seems to put a lot of time and effort into the deception. Is it less expensive to dupe than to recoup? It is like insurance companies, who seem to spend more money on finding ways to not pay a claim than it would cost them to just pay the claim. I have seen tiny little spaces used as patients' hospital rooms through which JACHO had passed through and stated 'the room is not even big enough to be a closet' (some exaggeration for effect—I hope). The hospital administrators make the arrangements in following inspections to move the patient, who is in the room, out, while the inspectors come through and yet, after a brief period post-inspection, the patient, like the empty beds in the hallways, finds themselves back in the room not fit to be a closet. Go figure.

Space is at a premium in some of these older hospitals in today's healthcare environment. Space is money. I've worked in rooms that are so tight for space that the overly obese nurse (and they are in the majority here in the Northeast) cannot even get around the bed to do proper patient care.

On other levels the cleanliness of floors, walls, and patient rooms, along with nurses stations miraculously and incredibly improves just prior to the inspection. Floors are glistening and sparklingly clean; elevators shine like new. I suppose it is not a bad thing to have a 'spring' cleaning every three to five years but really, it is shameful for a hospital to harbor such filth in-between times.

One can only imagine how many more improprieties abound behind the curtains of which I have not stepped.

THE UNIVERSE

Dealing with death on a regular basis—there are times where the ICU has sent sometimes four or five patients to the morgue in a 12-hour shift—and regularly manipulating life on a molecular level, sometimes with good results, sometimes not, brings about a slightly different view, perhaps, of the universe as a whole, for some.

The universe, as has been said in the past, of 'human expression,' is most certainly "unfolding as it should." Energy of suns breaks down all things, animate and inanimate alike, in its subtle ways. The human experience and, for that matter (pun by happenstance), life itself, in all its varied and vast ways, now and for some time, will continue in its cycle of itself until, by continuity, it will wear itself down, and all will be added to the entropy: chaos. The energy from suns reduces all to base form, which, at some point in time, is just another abstract along with all the other illusions of the bio-existence, for there is no, as some like to think, beginning and end. To use a phrase: "it just is." Sure, from a human standpoint there is beginnings and endings but this is shortsighted. The forces of nature are cyclical and rhyme; are harmonious and rhythmic. Once all matter is reduced to its elemental form, the force of energy is reduced, or expanded if you like, to, what we humans are now calling black holes of the universe. Black holes that have a great draw for all matter of the universe, as we know it. When base matter enters this "black hole," the forces within increase, or decrease, drawing more to it until even lesser black holes are gobbled up and expand exponentially beyond human comprehension until all of the entire universe and beyond is sucked into one complete being that some might like to equate to God, or the Truth; Wisdom or Justice. Call it what you will. Nothing is static; all is dynamic. Once the truth is known, it expands into a force so great that the "Big Bang" ensues, again, and casts its super-charged elements back outward into the unknown emptiness to fill it again anew, to reform, collect, and take shape from spinning and hurling to form into new existence other beings. Whether it is carbon-based, with the utilization of O2 for energy, or some other arrangement—it need not matter what configuration, really, for the energy itself begins the cycle again to wear itself down into elemental matter, which goes round and round, forever and ever. So what does this tell us? What is the purpose of life? No purpose at all. It just is. This, of course, is my view. Take it or leave it. It is no matter.

Notwithstanding, there is good "karma" and bad "karma," but, all in all, once cast in stone, it takes longevity on the human observational side to wear it down. There really is no time in matter, but there is certainly matter in time, meaning: matter only finds itself in phases, to be repeated over and over again in different configurations, but the animate is a place in time, which can be equated to just about anything you want it to be, being the humans that we are. So this comes right down to Einstein's Theory of Relativity, as I have come to see it: perspective. It is all on perspective—how one sees a position from the position of which they themselves personally view. And keep in mind this can be external or internal. Many internalize matter, which really is no matter at all, and yet to them it is. So is it real or is it imagined? And then: does it even really matter? This is where, I believe, life gets murky, and the darkness can overwhelm those who choose to see things as a whole different light of the unknown, which we, here, among the living, like to call death. But really what is death but a morphing of the matter.

140

There is no time. There is no beginning and end. This is God. This is beyond all human comprehension. That is God. Beyond all human understanding; the black hole of existence, from where all things come and are to return, over and over again in one big cycle of universe. Expand and contract. That's it. Going with the flow whether you know it or not, whether you want to or not. No one gets out alive. We as humans just count energetic excitations of electrons to mark an arbitrary structure based on one particular star closest to us here on earth. So why bother, you might say? I say, why not? It is an amazing ride. Looking past all the human shortcomings, the biosphere itself is worth taking-in in this short time we have to do it in such a fashion as the human experience. In the glorification of the whole one might do well by striving for such. We are, as they say, "all connected." "One can only hope."

This then would certainly progress in the direction of explaining "yin and yang" of the world, as we know it. And yet, like stupid, no one can explain it, only observe.

STRANGE OCCURRENCES

One night, working in the medical ICU, I was going to take a break and eat my garden fresh tomato, as I often do when the season is ripe. As I'm walking past a patient's room, a couple of nurses standing at the foot of the patient's bed asked me if I could take a moment to go over some of the basic concepts of this fairly new mode of mechanical ventilation, called, by some: "Bi-Level," just beginning to be used in this hospital, being run on that patient. As I'm going over some of the nuances of this mode of ventilation a resident doctor, with whom I had just had a consult on another patient, comes into the room and asks me, "Do you have GERD?"

[GERD being an acronym for gastro-esophageal regurgitation disorder, of which, it is presumed, some acidic foods, like tomatoes, are thought to exacerbate symptoms.]

Just out of the blue she asks if I have GERD.

"What? Do I have GERD? Why would you ask me that?" I replied, surprised.

She says: "I see you're holding a tomato."

My honest reply to her was "No, I have never had an incident of heartburn until just a week or two ago, and now I have been getting these incapacitating heartburn attacks. I've resorted to taking Tums." This doctor never, that I remember, gave me any satisfactory answer as to why she asked me that.

Now I was curious. I started talking about it with my colleagues, some of whom, surprisingly I find out, had been experiencing similar recent bouts of heartburn as never before. And, like myself, only at work. Also, like myself, they tried to pass it off as induced by work-related stress. In the course of talking to people about this, I had mentioned it to the 'overly-ambitious' Respiratory supervisor and her immediate reply was: "You might want to go see your doctor. That can be a sign of a heart attack." Strange?

I cut out all types of foods that might be a factor, even my beloved tomatoes. I cut out coffee. I meditated. All to no avail! I was at a loss. Tums helped with some symptom relief. Then one day it was gone. No more incapacitating heartburn. Just gone. That's it. I went back to my favorite dressing of vinegar and fish sauce on rice with garden fresh tomatoes, hot peppers, raw garlic and ginger. The heartburn never, to this day, returned. Strange!

Another time, one night while I'm going about my rounds and, as always, being somewhat aware as to what is going on in the unit, I notice the curtain to one of the patient's rooms is drawn tightly closed. This is usually done if a patient has just passed and has yet to be packed up and sent down to the morgue, or maybe family are having a discussion about the difficult decisions they are in need of making, or maybe it is just a patient's need for some privacy— these rooms around the central nurses' station have no doors, and some not fit to be a "closet," as noted.

This night the curtain was closed for privacy, and the patient was not on my list for any respiratory services so I did not pay much attention but for the curtain being closed.

Then, at some point, early in the shift, the resident doctor on comes up to me and asks to have a blood gas (ABG) drawn on this patient, a young woman, human immunodeficiency virus (HIV) positive who, I found out later, contracted the disease coming through the birth canal 21 years ago. I draw the blood.

[A blood gas is when an arterial blood sample is taken—1cc is usually sufficient. The measurement of the gases within the arterial blood yields a lot of information in its own right and then even more when compared to other test results. With the blood gas results one looks at the partial pressures of oxygen (PaO2) and carbon dioxide (PaCO2) dissolved within the arterial blood, the pH of the blood, calculated bicarbonate (HCO3) and blood/oxygen saturations and other calculations.]

When I drew the gas on this particular patient, there were visitors in the room: Dad and his wife (not the girl's mom. The girl's mother—I found out later—died years ago from Anti-human Immuno-Deficiency Syndrome: AIDS). The patient was pleasant and talkative, seeming a little sedate, but, as I said, I had no knowledge of why this patient was even in the hospital, never mind the ICU. Most patients in an ICU have some type of sedative on board; being in the hospital can cause anxiety in its own right even in the most stable "rock-of-a-person" patient. So I didn't find any real cause for concern while conversing with this very pleasant young lady; she was cooperative and talkative and friendly.

[This institution that I speak of here, many times, will put patients in an ICU bed with overly exaggerated or even fictitious complaints or diagnoses just to fill out the census. They are all about extrapolating as much money out of the system as possible via the patient and the insurance companies or the Commonwealth tax payer, sometimes known as "third-party payers," as mentioned. This institution does not like empty beds, too much lost revenue potential. Direct patient care employees can very often tell which patient has a very good health insurance plan from those who may not. The ones with good insurance usually get a lot of testing and ordered attention. The only others who get such élite care are the hospital executives and their families and some such dignitaries and the ones who cannot pay at all but for the Commonwealth footing the bill. Padding makes for good cushions.]

This particular young patient was an easy "stick." I run the ABG test at the bedside with a handheld device that takes 120 seconds to completion. Sometimes, as Einstein would appreciate, these two minutes can appear to take forever. When the girl's results come up I see no flags that would indicate any inaccuracies in the results, but the extremely low pH jumps right out at me as one that is not conducive to life: 6.9. Her HCO3 is in the single digits, which tells me right away to suspect the kidneys are shutting down. She needs an increase in ventilation (breathing), to compensate quickly for the low buffer, by purging (blowing-off) as much of the acid (CO_2) as possible. Large breathes with a long exhalation time is needed to eliminate the CO_2. This, of course has its limits. A stat bicarbonate bolus would certainly need to be considered when the HCO3 is in single digits (Normal range being 22 to 26 mEq/L {some ranges vary}) to get the pH back on track. This girl is on death's door and about to die and die very quickly if intervention is not implemented immediately.

I did not know anything about this case at the time of the ABG drawing but for the fact that the doctor ordered the blood gas to be drawn. I didn't even know why the gas had been ordered. But, I knew immediately upon seeing the gas results that if I did not act quickly she would, with all probability, 'code' within minutes: cardiac arrest, and die. Muscles do not like acid, and the heart is a big bad muscle that, when in a rebellious mood, will just stop pumping and die if no remedial action is taken to get oxygen to its cells and correct the blood pH derangement. I ran and grabbed a stand-by Bi-Pap machine that we try to always have standing ready for such emergencies. Emergencies, as one can imagine, happen quite frequently in a medical/pulmonary ICU. (Working equipment however is very often in short supply; cutbacks directly affect pt. care when institutions direct more funds toward upper-management salaries.)

I quickly plugged in the oxygen and electrical lines of the Bi-Pap machine and put in emergent settings while informing the patient (the Dad and others visiting had stepped out of the room by this time) what I was doing as I was doing it and said, "we are going to use this machine with the mask to help you breathe." The girl looks up at me and says, in a very kind and gentle way: "I LOVE YOU." She looked right at me and said I love you. I didn't know what to say. I was not expecting such a statement. I didn't know her; she didn't know me. All I heard coming out of MY mouth was, "I love you, Honey." I couldn't believe, at this point, that she was even alive never mind talking. I placed the mask on her and was able to ventilate. 'Anesthesia' was called, came, intubated, and I placed the patient on the ventilator.

My emotions were reeling, I felt she must have seen me as her father, for it seemed to me her father was a loving and caring one who took good care of his daughter. He was there.

[Some patients, even on death's doorstep, never get a visitor at all. It must be unsettling, to say the least, to have to die among strangers. I really admire people who have loved ones surrounding them when they pass.]

I thought to myself at the time, and still like to believe, that her deranged metabolic state, which can cause confusion, resulted in a case of mistaken identity. I thought: "She must really come from a loving caring family to have, in such a life-changing moment such as this, love on her mind. I could not stop crying on the way home from work that night.

The next night when I showed up for work she was gone. Dead. I learned then about her biological mother having HIV, and how her father had witnessed the horrific sufferings of his wife at that time, this girl's mother, dying of AIDS.

Earlier in the day the dad had made the decision to withdraw care for his daughter. They did, and she died. Dad, I was told, said: "I watched my wife, her mother, suffer and die a long, drawn out, painfully suffering death. I will not put my daughter through that!"

God bless that man.

Another time working the medical "torture chamber" a young girl in her 20s comes in, and I'm requested to assess her trache due to bleeding and irritation. She is ventilated and with feeding tube. I come to find in her medical history that she is suffering from a rapid onset of Amyotrophic Lateral Sclerosis (ALS); a motor neuron disease also known as Lou Gehrig's disease. She has two little girls; by looking at them I guessed they were, at the time, around 5 and 3. This patient was very pleasant and concerned that the homecare she was getting from outside services was not adequate—to be polite—causing trauma to her trachea, thus the bleeding. This is not uncommon. People who are medically trained, even within the hospital setting itself, are not comfortable with traches and cause a lot of unnecessary pain and suffering, even damage to the patient and their airway out of lack of care and/or concern (aka: laziness) or just downright apathy or ignorance.

Her husband, or boyfriend/children's father, or just boyfriend, I didn't really know, was there and very supportive. He, too, was young; they were around the same age.

She spent a few days and nights with us in the ICU, and her trache was healing up nicely; the bleeding stopped and irritation relieved.

On one of these particular nights I'm talking with her nurse at the nurses' station just outside this girl's room and all of a sudden "**BOOM**" from this patient's room. The nurse and I run into the room and find the patient's partner, the young man, passed out on the floor. He is lying over the IV lines, which were running from the IV pump on an IV pole next to the bed to the pt. The nurse and I didn't know what had transpired, but the boy was "out-cold" lying on the floor. The helpless patient looked panic-stricken and petrified, fear in her eyes, unable to do anything herself to help, for she had no use of any bodily functions. She couldn't even call for help.

This young girl, who, just a short time ago I imagine, was living a healthy, vibrant life, is now in need of total and constant care. She cannot breathe on her own; she has no movement of any limbs; others must meet all her activities of daily living (ADL's); she had no way of taking care of herself at this point, never mind taking care of others, like her little girls. Very stressful, to say the least!

For some reason (I will never know) she decided to check out. I do not mean AMA and leave the hospital for home; she had lost her will to live. I suppose she had lost hope. I do not know how the decision was made and who was involved, but the doctor wrote the order to discontinue all supportive care.

Watching the two little girls walk down that hallway and enter their mom's room for their very last goodbyes was beyond heart wrenching. The young mom was removed from the ventilator, the feeding tube discontinued, and she was pronounced dead shortly thereafter. And again, fighting back tears on my ride home reflecting on the events, I find myself asking: "Where's the God in that? Where?"

THE DOCTOR

Behind most every doctor there seems to be a very big ego (maybe there needs to be)—I may exaggerate some to make the point.

Doctors today do some amazing health miracles no doubt but we all have our limitations. People in this society will abuse themselves with very poor lifestyle choices for 20, 30 and even 40 years or so and then, when internal systems begin to fail and their health becomes compromised beyond the point of ignoring it, will call on the doctor and expect to be "fixed-up good-as-new" in two weeks.

To be fair one must acknowledge there are certain types of people that can be categorized and classified on many levels, not least the psychological, which group certain types into professions. Doctors are ones with huge egos. Doctors, especially young ones right out of medical school, seem to think they must present themselves as all-knowing. With these doctors, ego trumps objectivity every time. These doctors will not listen to reason or rationale. They must know all. They are the doctors; everyone must listen to, and believe, and do, what they say, right or wrong. This, objectively, is absolute lunacy. Allied health professionals learn quite a bit from years of experience working in the live laboratory. When a doctor, just out of medical school, condescends to a nurse, who has, let's say, 30-plus years of experience working in an ICU, the doctor makes himself or herself look really bad. It is the doctor who works with the other members of the team to improve the health and wellbeing of a patient that earns deserved respect from team members and colleagues and pt.'s alike.

I'll say it again: arrogance is really just a mask ignorance hides behind. Doctors are very good at this. Physicians condescending and intimidating other professionals in a show of superiority to quell dissention and keep people on their knees has cost many patients their lives—usually not before much pain and suffering.

The medical/pulmonary ICU, in which I worked for many years, became known as the "torture chamber" (as stated above) for all the immoral and unethical things done to patients all at the order of the doctor. If the doctor orders it, you must do it or else. Or else what, you may ask? Or else you are out of a job. Staff torture patients when the staff member fears job loss. They will do anything to keep their job; they'll sell their souls. Remember most everyone has his or her price. It is a sad state of affairs. And then, when you throw at them: "What if that was your parent?" Many do not hold up to the moral dilemma.

I view doctors like the conductor of an orchestra; they are at the head of all the instruments and players and have a grand overview of the whole. The doctor conducts the care of the patient by gathering information from each ancillary medical discipline and pieces together the puzzle of the illness via first a diagnosis and cause, then a plan, and, hopefully, with any luck, a cure. Each "player" is instrumental to the whole ensemble yet only sees from a limited viewpoint within the body as a whole. The doctor is the one who has all the information and the one to bring the piece to a harmonious conclusion.

These days however doctors seem to have become the drug pushers with a license to steal...a license to kill? Not premeditated but, in my view, irresponsible. "Manslaughter" in their quest for the almighty dollar? Not all, but certainly a good number of medical professionals these days are in the trade to make money. The days when a doctor went into medicine to help reduce suffering and find a cure are well behind us.

It is sad, in a very pathetic way, to watch doctors struggle with their egos. I'll give you an example. In the RR, responding to a respiratory distress emergency call, the respiratory therapist finds a post-op patient who is unresponsive. Possibly due to over-sedation from surgery (this happens often) or excess fluid in the lungs—the "OR" likes to hydrate for surgery, sometimes too much.

[Excess fluid can settle in the lungs: pulmonary edema: drowning from within.]

Over sedation is not an uncommon occurrence when too much sedation for a surgery causes prolonged intubation and mechanical ventilation while waiting for the drugs to metabolize (wear off) and the patient to wake up. This patient, on this particular call, appeared to have been extubated too soon; sedation was still having an effect and the patient's respirations were shallow, weak, and ineffective to sustain life. The airway was patent, and the patient was easily ventilated with bag and mask. The anesthesiologist, however, wanted to reintroduce the "breathing tube," and proceeded to intubate. Not bad practice *per se.* The more appropriate question would be on the decision to extubate when they did.

The intubation appeared to be difficult right from the start.

[Once an ET tube is introduced (inserted) the therapist along with doctors and nurses, per protocol, check for tube placement to ensure it is in fact in the trachea (airway) leading to the lungs and not in the esophagus leading to the stomach. Placement is checked by several methods. One being a very quick and easy bedside check with a very simple device called an "end tidal CO_2 detector." This "detector" has a "gas-sensitive" mesh that changes color from blue to gold in the presence of CO_2. The gaseous exposure upon exhalations brings about this color change— gold is good—which gives an indication of the presence of CO_2 in the expired gas or, with no change in color, a lack thereof. The sensor is placed in between the ET tube and the "Ambu bag" (manual respirator) and given a few breaths, watch for pt. chest rise, and look for color change in the detector. Simple, easy, and accurate. As the exhaled air flows through the mesh in the sensor it will detect CO_2, which is in large concentrations in the exhaled gas of the lungs. Color change indicates the tube is in the right place: the trachea. This color change must be consistent and continuous. It is recommended to see color change on five consecutive breaths, assuring confidence the tube is in "the lungs." The stomach sometimes may contain CO_2 and could initially create a gold color change, but this will not last. Once the CO_2 content of the stomach is purged, color change ceases.

It is also protocol to auscultate, with a stethoscope, the chest and belly—listening for air movement and noting whether there is anatomical differentiation more pronounced over the lungs or stomach, if at all. This can help indicate whether the trachea or esophagus has been "tubed."

The final check on tube placement is with a portable chest x-ray. This, however, takes some time to have the portable x-ray machine to the room, shoot the film, and then back to the x-ray department for development. This is to check tube depth—where the tube is in relation to the vocal cords and the carina.

Generally the tip of the ET tube should be just above the carina (the bifurcation of the trachea into the right and left main-stem bronchi) about three centimeters.]

In this particular case, once the ET tube was inserted and checked for placement with the End Tidal CO2 detector, all medical staff present was able to see that there was no color change. No good breath sounds were heard within the thoracic chest area. Clearly the tube was not a conduit to the lungs. The O2 saturation monitor continued in a downward trend, meaning poorly oxygenated blood, another objective indicator of improper placement of the ET tube.

The belly continued to distend. The anesthesiologist doctor insisted he had the tube in the trachea. The respiratory therapist on the scene refuted this assessment as to the objectivity that indicated the tube was not in the trachea and "the tube should be pulled." The doctor insisted the tube was in, but could not deny the severe gravity of the objective deteriorating condition of this patient at this time. He, the doctor, who was at the head of the bed refused to pull the tube out and ventilate via "bag and mask," which had proven successful prior. Good effective ventilation with manual resuscitation bag and mask is possible with almost everyone. The only problem with this maneuver is fatigue of the manual "ventilator": the one holding the "bag."

Instead, the doctor intubating in this case decided to leave the one tube, which was clearly in the esophagus, in—all could clearly see that at this point the patient's belly was so full of air it looked like it was ready to burst like a balloon. When the belly was depressed, all could hear the air passing back out the tube. The doctor made another attempt to insert another ET tube into the trachea, which by this time must have been severely narrowed by the other tube occupying the esophagus, thus depressing or flattening the trachea to deformity and collapse, or near collapse at the very least, making it almost impossible, I imagine, to pass another tube. When, in medical emergencies, things go "south" (go bad), they go south very fast! This was not going well, and now had two ET tubes, with no "color-change," going into the esophagus and nothing allowing for ventilation of the lungs, thus depriving this patient of vital life sustaining oxygen: asphyxiation by suffocation. Without oxygen to the living cell, the cell dies very fast.

Cardiac arrest came soon for this poor soul who, upon putting his faith in the medical profession, possibly there for a routine day-procedure, suffocated at the hands of the egocentric modern doctor. The patient cardiac arrested; chest compressions promptly ensued—in an exercise of futility, for it is of no good use to get blood circulating if it is carrying no oxygen. After an extended period of frantic, pathetically masked heroics to save this poor man's life, he was pronounced dead. Due to the gravity of a routine surgery gone bad, so to speak, the Anesthesia Attending was called to the bedside while the corpse was still warm, to assess the situation. As soon as he arrived, he asked if there had been a color change on the CO_2 detector. The doctors involved gave an immediate "yes." Which was an outright lie. The therapist standing along side the doctor at the beds head, without hesitation, chimed in that "NO, it did not. Two times!" The Attending used fiber optics and confirmed what was already known: both ET tubes were in the esophagus. This was the end of the story for respiratory therapy's role in the event and the end of the pt. What the doctors told the family is possibly another story all together.

On another case, at another time, respiratory therapy was called to an emergent respiratory-distress situation in the "short-stay" area, where patients are also brought for routine day procedures. Upon arrival there was a female anesthesiologist tending to a pt. on a gurney who appeared in great distress; in a state of anxiety. I am not aware of the circumstances that led up to "Respiratory" being called but when the respiratory therapist arrived the patient was breathing on his own. His respiratory rate was high—to be expected in cases of severe anxiety/panic attack—yet his oxygenation was good. However, for some reason, other than to assume the doctor's mantra: "airway protection", "Anesthesia" (the doctor) was determined to intubate to secure the airway.

This is not out of the realm of good medical practice. She, the anesthesiologist, administered drugs that aid in the process of introducing the ET tube. Sometimes paralytics are a drug of choice of the anesthesiologists allowing passing of the tube into the trachea more accommodating — presumably.

[I, for one, am not a big proponent of paralyzing a patient who is breathing on his or her own. If the airway has yet to be secured and the intubation attempt fails, the patient is still at least ventilating, moving air, and oxygenating to some degree on his or her own accord. Paralytics can be a double-edged sword; for if the tube cannot be passed easily "through the chords" (vocal chords) you now have a patient that cannot breathe, for the paralytics have rendered the muscles of the respiratory system useless. And, what's worse, if appropriate sedatives are not administered in conjunction, the pt. is totally aware of what is going on around them, and yet, cannot do a single thing to save him or herself, like breathe.]

This patient was now in a severe state of anxiety/panic attack, which was reflected in his heart rate and blood-pressure, which was, by this time (as they say behind the curtain) "through the roof." The anesthesiologist was insistent on intubating this patient but "could not pass the tube." The patient was deteriorating quickly. "LMA's save lives" (Laryngeal Mask Airway) was suggested to the anesthesiologist doctor, who dismissed it for reasons I can only conjecture. EGO? When the doctor finally realized that the whole team was questioning her ability to secure an airway and repeated proclamations of "LMA's save lives" she finally acquiesced. But to no avail, this institution, at that time, did not stock their "CODE carts" with LMA's. Nor did this anesthesiologist have one in her bag. It was known that there were some in the ER, so one ran to get one. By the time the LMA arrived the patient was already gone. He had cardiac arrested and died. A simple outpatient procedure and the patient dies! What do you tell the family? "The doctor knows best?" Let the buyer beware.

There have been CODE's where the doctor, having been handed the bedside blood gas results, reads off the range values printed on the slip thinking they were the actual patient's results. The doctor thought the CODE team was doing a wonderful job at reviving this patient with "text book" gas results. The doctor had to be redirected to the actual results, which were not so stellar.

WHEN GOD CALLS

"Your time is up"; "End of the line"; "Piper wants to be paid," Whichever mantra one may choose, the concept is the same: you do not have a choice when "your time is up." When called to death, one will obey, like it or not. Oh sure, modern medicine has bought some people some additional years and even improved the quality of life for many I dare say, being a blessing to some family and friends still among the living. For many others, though, it's just a prolongation of suffering.

One evening early, while working the ER trauma room, a call comes in that an "electrocution" was on its way in. A lineman, working up in a bucket-lift, some like to call a "cherry-picker," stood up and hit his head on a live wire. The electricity entered through his skull, causing a gaping open-wound there at the top of his head. As the electricity traveled to ground it blew both his eyes out and then the electrical current exited his right hand where another wound was found. And, to add insult to injury, in real terms, the electrical current was such a shock it flipped his body out of the bucket, which was said to be 30 feet up in the air, hurling him down to the ground below.

When he got to the ER he was not in good shape. His eyes, after the bandages were removed, could be seen charred and hanging out. His brain tissue was oozing and hanging out of his skull, and his right hand was the least of his worries. Intubation was done in the field, so vitals and the physical assessment were done quickly in the ER and x-rays were taken while a quick job of rewrapping the head wounds was performed to keep tissue from exposure and flopping around as much as possible to get him up to the OR. Per protocol, a CT scan was the next stop on the way to the OR.

Amazingly, this big burly man, the pt., while sliding him over onto the CT scanner table, wakes up and starts thrashing around like he's at a National Wrestlers Championship meet. Unable to see, the bandages upon his head and eyes flying loose in his frantic attempt to get up, brain and eye tissue flinging side to side as his head is thrashing wildly. The doctor grabs his head to try to stabilize it and hold some of the dressings in place to save tissue, while another holds his jaw and ET tube to keep the airway in place. It took three others to try to hold him down on this very narrow scanner table. Frantically requesting sedation, the nurse, scrambling to find them, realized the sedation meds were left in the ER from which the pt. and staff had so quickly exited to get to the OR via CT scanner.

Mayhem ensued. Other staff members in the radiology department, hearing the commotion, came and lent their hands, and body weight, to keep this patient down, who was very insistent on going against staff's wishes. Someone called down to the ER requesting meds: "STAT!"

Finally sedation came, the CT scan was done, and the pt. was transported to the OR and eventually placed in the trauma ICU.

It was a long and painful recovery I would imagine, but recover he did, amazingly. Blinded, and with some brain damage no doubt, but alive and being discharged after a very long, extended stay, as one could imagine; from ICU to the Floors, then to discharge—probably to a rehab facility. I did lose track of this patient once he was off of respiratory care services but would hear at times, much to my amazement, how well he was doing.

The last I heard of him he was being discharged from the hospital—he was there about six to eight months—and, on his way out the door to a rehab facility, while sitting in the wheelchair, the "Piper" demanded to be paid: the patient cardiac arrested and died, right then and there, after all that.

On other levels; when the decision is made to move from life to death one tries to come to grips with the reality that circumstances change, and sometimes, in my view, it is more humane to let someone go: die, instead of prolonging suffering. The hardest thing in life sometimes, however, is to let go of a loved one – as I'm sure many can imagine, or already know. It seems like an easy concept, but really, for most, it is not. Hospice has the tools and experience in dealing with the transition.

Watching someone die is a very humbling experience. I have observed, over the years, many people die; people who seem to have a strong faith in God meet death, more often than not, with grace and dignity. Those without move in panic and fear. Sorry to say.

Nevertheless, one never really knows unless going down that road. Here's an example: One Thanksgiving around 20:00 we get word from the ER that a 93-year-old male pt. is coming up to the unit after choking on some turkey at dinner. The ER therapist gives report: "Family activated 911; performed CPR for about 10 minutes before EMS arrived; unresponsive upon arrival; vitals stable; intubated in the field for airway protection; ventilated and stable. Blood Gas: 7.48/33/212/22/100%. I turned the rate down. We'll see you in a few minutes. We're in CT now and will be heading up as soon as we're through. See you then."

Why would EMS intubate a 93-year-old one might ask: To keep him alive for months on end to drain the coffers while the pt. now tortured and rots in the bed?

By 05:00 hours the next day, less than 24 hours from the incident, we have the pt. extubated. As soon as the tube comes out he says, "Can I see my girlfriend?" This gentleman's number, for now, must have been unlisted in the heavens.

Medicine is a tough vocation; it is sad it has been overtaken by business.

The only one to really skirt death, we are told, is Enoch: the one who "walked" with God. There must be something in this story that runs deeper than most humanity. There must be something in this that instructs us about death. Certainly, most of us anyway, would not believe this story on the face of it, or would have a hard time with it at least, except for the true fanatic, who has a hard time with life as a whole, and needs something to lean on. The Bible can be a good crutch, but one needs to remember a crutch is something to help us along, to help us along the path we have chosen for ourselves when folly turns us into fools. So what does Enoch have to teach us about death? Maybe nothing. For what would he know? He never experienced death we are told. Or so it is written. Heuristics is what teaches hard lessons in life, so why would death be any different? Only to experience death firsthand can we come to know it intimately and completely.

SOCIAL STRUCTURE

The whole social structure has begun to feed on itself. The healthcare industry is just that, an industry. The production of goods and services, in all its many facets, is making us sick and in need of health care. And Healthcare steps in. Albeit Healthcare is close to the number one employer of the communities it serves and these days are making good money at it. Much like the government, it grows into this unstoppable beast. It continues to spread, almost as if feeding on itself. But in reality it feeds off of the taxpayer: the hard working class; the proletariat. GDP is some closely watched number some feel needs to advance at all cost. Time and again when truth comes to light we find duplicity. Our whole social and economic structure has come to the point where we need lots of sickly people (which we do have) in need of health care, again "Healthcare" steps in to take the charge, provide care, and, in the same vain, keeps much of the community employed, bills paid, and benefits funded. Just like government bureaus, which never seem to die, keep a lot of people out of the unemployment lines. Which is where, by the way, nursing, as a career, is promoted because "it pays well."

The system of healthcare is feeding on itself. Healthcare is making the employee sick with poor working conditions coupled with poor nutrition. Oh sure they say, "We promote healthy diets, healthy lifestyles" and then close down the cafeteria at night and stock the vending machines with sweet/salty snacks chockfull of chemicals that the body does not readily recognize and so instantly turns it into storage/fat. It does not take long for a new nurse just out of nursing school, taking a night job, to pack on the pounds. It takes its toll over the years. The stress, as studies have shown, takes its toll. The studies are out there. At some point the caregiver becomes the patient. And the "bottom-line" people find it all very convenient. After all, the institutions of Healthcare/hospitals pay a lot of money to the health insurance industry and the government throughway of premiums and taxes of which they want to recoup. What better way than replacing the herd with younger, less expensive workers while the older workers are sent out to pasture and become the new "cash-cow" of the day with all their health issues now in need of health care.

When all hope is gone, life ceases to exist for many. Without hope we have nothing. Is not God really an exercise in faith and hope? When a person loses all hope, death soon comes. With the fear of losing hope we see desperate acts. Acting out of frustration people will go to extreme measures. People will lash out at anything that threatens their life, be it real or imagined, petty or fleeting. If the one in desperation feels threatened, they lash out, many times in violent ways. This is the "carrot-*on*-the-stick" phenomenon. Always just out of reach. This is the "haves-and-have-nots" syndrome. At some point the "mule" gets tired and just gives up; lost is all hope of achieving the goal. That is the capitalist society in which we live, in the Occident, in this "Western" world. Eventually, I would dare say, many come to a point in their lives and are forced, whether they like it or not, to face the very real fact that many, if not all, of their hopes and dreams, their aspirations and desires in life have not, and will not, be fulfilled. Many people deal with such revelations in many different ways. Many are just too old and tired to give a damn. Bitterness ensues. Depression is not uncommon. Suicides increase, when, as I have said, all hope is lost. Mass shootings! Kids killing kids! This comes about when being inundated by the media with all

the things they tell us we must have, indeed: need—
"can't-live-without" types of goods that really do
nothing in any measure to enhance our lives, and all
the while we must eventually pay to have all the
"shit," they told us we just had to have, taken away.
They are just like the stockbroker: they have you
paying on the way in and then paying again on the
way out. And yet we believe what they tell us. If you
work hard, you can have all this. Yet, there is the
carrot. There is always something better, something
newer, something some other glitterati have that we
do not, now feeling compelled that this, too, we must
have. "Does the pretty, young, sexy girl come with the
car?" For the price, one might imagine they would or
should. And yet, at home, late at night, quiet and still,
awakened with a hollow feeling inside, something is
not right. Something is not there; something is
missing! This all from Ado; from glorifying those who
are more blessed with a particular talent that is
viewed at the time as desirable and coveted, for
whatever reasons, which some place more
importance on than another.

Each to their vocation and to each a living
wage. Is this too much to ask of the community? We,
as a community, as a society, need to generate dignity
and respect to all, as all deserve to be treated with
equal dignity and respect. This is no new concept. As
a matter of fact, in a matter of speaking, this concept
is as "old-as-the-hills." It is not an easy system to
implement, for with power comes corruption; and in
a system of people someone has to make decisions,
and that is the one who has control over others. Only
a very strong resolve, with which very few have been
blessed over history's great breath of human
endeavors, will pass the test. The road is narrow,
with many "snakes" along the way (not to give snakes
a bad name, for they deserve better), the top exposed
and precarious, of which many cannot stand, but it is
the goal for which to strive. Without hope of a noble

goal and direction we are doomed to hopelessness, and I have shown where this leads. We, as a community, as a society, as a culture here in the 'First world' are headed in that direction but as of yet have not reached the true state of hopelessness. We are, however, close. We are in the phase of fear in losing hope and have become desperate as a society, not knowing which way to turn from lack of leadership and role models and irresponsible marketing by business for profits only, and now many are violently lashing out. What kind of a people, what kind of society has children mass killing children? Something is fundamentally wrong. It is the manifestation of a society that praises one and kicks another. A society of "haves" and "have-nots" where the "nots" are becoming tired, disillusioned, frustrated and disgusted that some "haves" so callously flaunt in the faces of the "have-nots" who have "not." No '**one**' can change this tide but '**everyone**' can.

And then again: Is there really something fundamentally wrong or are we passing through the phase set out by the universe unfolding as it must? The journey for humans, all life for that matter, is ambiguous, God holding all the cards of which we as humans are not privy to see the whole deck; the big black hole of the unknown. Now is the time to change tack. It is destiny.

Parenting has taken a toll on our social structure today. As children move through adolescence and puberty, their innocent years turned upside down by the introduction of hormones, which have life-changing effects, it is no wonder they lash out on many levels and in so many ways, out of frustration I suppose, when they find out their parents, along with so many others, have been lying to them for years.

I'll give you a brief list: Santa Claus; the Easter Bunny; the Tooth Fairy; the Sandman... the list goes on. Why, when the truth begins to surface about Santa Claus, would any young person trust the one who pushed the dupe? Not only does the young adult come to realize that his/her parents have been lying to them all this time but, on top of this revelation, is the realization that there is no nice guy who comes once a year, in the middle of the night, no less, to bring free gifts of all types and, in many cases, the very ones you have been coveting all year long. Why? Because they told you, is this why? And you trusted. Why? Because they told you to trust them! Duped! And to confuse the issues even more, the people in your life, who have been drilling into your head for years on end, know these lies, the ones who are supposed to be unfailingly trustworthy, are not. Who does the teen turn to then? When in-need most of confidential truth, where to turn? The Church, too, I am sad to say, have failed the community greatly over the years. Frustration ensues and violence, very often, erupts. And the parents, for the life of them, cannot figure out where they went wrong. All year long the parent teaches the little ones not to talk to strangers, "do not take candy from a stranger, stay away from strangers and do not let strangers into the house"; and yet, at Christmas time, they throw the children at this big, fat strange man with big white irritating facial hair, dressed in a strange red suit who is going to be allowed to come into the house at night when everyone is asleep. How confusing is that?

Why do we do it? Because of marketing, that is why. The history of "Santa Claus" is vast and varied, but one cannot refute the persona of commercialism the character has now taken on. Industrialization has created the monster, and the monster wants to be fed. The monster does not care about honesty and truth. The monster only cares about feeding the machine and how it affects the bottom line on the accountant's ledger. There are profits to be made, but at whose expense? Ultimately the culture and its social structure pay the price. It is very difficult to not over-indulge in the land-of-plenty. Discipline is in short supply when there are profits to be made. This is why we have government: to rein in the unscrupulously greedy.

Two-family incomes have also played a significant role in the cultural development of this social structure we live in here today in these United States of America entering the 21st century. The 30-year mortgage is not some arbitrary thing. Neither is hourly wages. It is a very structured system to consume a lifetime. Now I believe it is good to keep the masses busy on projects that enhance the lives of all within the commonwealth, but not at their expense by usury rates so that others can lord it over the many to their individual accumulation of wealth. One must remember that wealth, in economic terms, is just the control and distribution, or the divvying-up, if you will, of surpluses. The birth of surplus was the opening of the floodgates to greed. Was that the plan?

The American Founding "Farmers" knew well the meaning of the phrase "we reap what we sow." When sowing tobacco, or cotton or corn or what have you, the farmer is hopeful of his seed to yield a harvest. The "Farmers" built a society on agriculture. Living close to nature, to the land, early Americans had a different perspective on life than we today. Living in a plastic disposable world turned recycled, as many are today, can make for some crazy distorted shapes when exposed to heat. When the truth is masked in delusions to the ego, many run for the mundane thinking it adds quality to life.

This is the issue today, defining "quality of life"! Quality of life can be a very subjective display of emotion. If important life decisions are based on emotion, we run the risk of making bad choices in life.

We, as a community, need to be asking the question: Will the proposed procedure improve one's quality of life? One should be asking: Where is the improvement in quality of life? Many times we see the surgeon pushing the patient toward the operating suite when the outcome is questionable to make a difference in the patient's life quality. It's all about the money today. When is enough, enough? Surgeons like to cut. You go to a surgeon for medical advice, nine times out of 10 their solution to the problem is to cut; you go to a nutritionist, they will cure your ills by the foods you eat. This is all generalization and, of course, as we all know, there are exceptions to every rule, but the general trend of the professions nowadays is to make money. We all have bills to pay it is true. But there is a difference between working to make money and practicing a vocation.

We need a better plan. A big problem today in the medical field is family members/health care proxies who are not prepared to make such life-changing decisions. Many people think they are prepared for death when, in fact, when the time comes, they are shocked at just how unprepared they really are. The people who are dying and the loved ones at the bedside alike! People with emotional attachments do not, very often, make good healthcare proxies; they generally do not make good medical decisions based on objectivity. This is why people put their trust in the doctor. The doctor, some doctors, those who should be emotionally detached and are supposed to be making good ethically based decisions for the patients and families wellbeing, when the family's emotions are running high, are breaching that trust. The question becomes: Are we really focused on patient-centered care or doctor-centered care—or even institution-centered care? The problems being that the general population, with no knowledge of what really is going on medically, are being duped into trusting someone whose priorities have become askew. The doctor of today many times makes decisions on protecting him/herself from malpractice lawsuits and now are the tools making decisions on generating revenue. So who is truly advocating for the patient's best interest and their quality of life? Emotional family members can make for bad decisions. This is where Hospice needs to come in.

Mandate Hospice

CRASFTMAN-SHIFT

I believe the community would benefit greatly if statutes were on the books requiring hospitals and other healthcare facilities to be mandated to have Hospice care involved whenever anyone over the age of, say, 70 enters an ER or any medical facilities admissions office for any health or medical reason. Not only the patient but family members need to be educated as to what's to come, and given the tools that may help them get through the difficult time of saying their last goodbye's to a loved one. Too many times I've seen patients kept alive and suffer, unnecessarily in my view, so some family member can fly in from "kingdom come" and say goodbye to their loved one. They think this is showing love but really it is, in my view, very often a feeble attempt to purge guilt one last time; a miserably failing attempt to right all past wrongs. How cruel; and the doctors' grant the request and ancillary tortures, per doctors orders, until the "loved" one comes and says, "Ok, goodbye. Pull the plug." Sometimes it is just as pathetically cold as that.

Hospice, in my view, is an organization trained to objectify the realities of death in a kind and caring way. Hospice teaches those who are terminal and at the end of their lives, from whatever causes, if time allows, what to expect in the remaining time breathing on this earth. Not only teaching the patient what is to come and keeping them comfortable but also teaching the family members what may be expected. In my view this process is started much too late, and it is my firm belief that this educational process, of which, sooner or later, one way or another, we all come to learn, would be best started and expanded at an earlier age in life for all. We need to, as a community, start educating people sooner about the throes of death, what to expect, how things will play out, and how best to deal with it for ourselves, and our loved ones. This, for me, is truly patient-centered care. When life and death decisions need to be made, they need to be made with the dying person's best interest taken first and foremost. Too many times the family member makes decisions based on their deep-rooted emotional state that can be a quagmire of confusion or, even worse, fears played on by the doctors for business' sake. Guilt plays a huge role. Many people are not prepared to say their last goodbyes to a loved one, and so, unwittingly, on many occasions, prolong the suffering of their very own loved ones, the ones they are supposed to protect from suffering, yet just add to it and prolong, unnecessarily, the sufferings at times.

Start the educational process before death is cast upon us. Family members are not good at making these decisions because they have very little knowledge, if any at all, on how to deal with a loved one dying.

So what happens today more often than not? The patients are institutionalized/hospitalized for extended periods of time. Family member not ready to make the decision to let a loved one go and the institution, seeing dollar signs, uses fear mongering mixed with just the right amount of hopeless-hope to extend the stay for revenue purposes only. They want to spend all the money before the opportunity is lost, aka: when the patient dies. Healthcare has developed into a stealthily underhanded abusive relationship with the community. First making people sick, under the guise of GDP, feeding them a bunch of shit to the point of bursting along the "First-World" order of a sedentary life style, which has almost all

170

brainwashed into coveting the illusion of a "good life." People flock to the United States to get "fat." Then, once sick and in need of a cure, the medical profession offers plenty of treatments to ease the suffering—which only helps ease for a time. Please don't get me wrong, I'm all for the easing of suffering—yet very seldom does the medical profession offer any real cure. Where's the profit in curing?

Relieve symptoms and "see me in a week." "Keep them sick, but keep them alive." This is healthcare today in the 21st century.

Even the craftsman today, who builds to last—unless in an expanding population—knows all too well they will find themselves out of work and in the unemployment lines in a very short order.

WE TAKE CARE OF OUR OWN

Now, if you don't mind, I will give a little personal account of my own experience as a patient. Skin cancer has been a problem in my family and has become an issue for me over the years. Being, at the time, employed by this large institution, I was fortunate (or not) to have very good health insurance coverage. I, along with my father, have been 'diagnosed' with several kinds of skin cancer: basal cell, squamous cell, and metastatic melanoma. My father died from, among other issues, another malignant typed skin cancer: Merkel cell.

After having my first diagnosis of basal cell carcinoma on my back removed I was recommended to have checkups at the dermatology clinic every six months, which I did. Usually they would not find anything of great concern, but, as one oncologist came to observe: "they are always freezing something"—referring to spraying a growth on the skin with CO_2 to freeze it, and then eventually it falls off. This is done on very benign growths. Sometimes they might find a growth of concern, cut it off and send it to the lab for analysis.

One night, at work, I had made a quick exit from the sixth floor ICU torture chamber to use the toilet. On my way out the doubled metal fire doors, going from the main hospital to the medical school section of the institution, where bathrooms are located, the large metal plate at the top edge of the door, used to lock the doors automatically magnetically, came loose and, in a deadfall, crashed down into my right forearm, leaving a bloody gash. Made of iron about three-quarters of an inch thick and maybe eight inches by four inches—a very heavy steel plate—must have come loose by extended use and lack of maintenance. Supervisors and Employee Health were notified and made light of the incident. I continued to work. After some time of healing I had forgotten about the incident and carried on with my work and life.

At some point after this incident, about four or five months, I, and my little boy, noticed a small round-shaped bump rising up from the site where the injury from the metal plate had occurred, with a very purplish discoloration; it looked like the top of a worn-down pencil eraser in shape and size. I didn't think much of it except for the fact that I would find myself picking at it unconsciously from time to time. It did not bleed. I had, at this point forgotten all about the trauma to my arm in the very same spot.

With my family history of skin cancer I brought this growth to the attention of the nurse practitioner on my six-month visit at the dermatology clinic.

She, the nurse practitioner, disregarded visually this new growth as a "keratosis," a benign skin growth, of which I've had a few. She did, however, come up with some basal cell on my scalp, which I had surgically removed at a later set appointment. All went well with the basal cell removed from my scalp, but the growth on my arm kept growing. I felt I was in need of a closer observation—my dad died from the Merkel cell carcinoma that had developed on his leg. The bump on my arm kept getting larger, and my five-year-old son kept questioning it with: "what's that bump on your arm?" It was by now about the size of a new unused pencil erasure in its height. On my next six-month check-up at the same clinic with the same nurse I requested it be removed for biopsy. I had to insist. The nurse practitioner was still not concerned but did remove it for biopsy at my insistence. Usually dermatology looks with great adventure at cutting things off of me. I was somewhat baffled at her hesitation to take a biopsy. Anyway, she did and the biopsy report came in from the lab: metastatic melanoma.

As soon as the nurse practitioner got the lab results she called me immediately and left a message to call her back right away. The message was to have her come to the phone even to be interrupted if she was with another patient when I called. I knew right away what news I was about to get with a message like that. Not very often will a health care professional tell a secretary to interrupt a patient office visit for a phone call. It is usually: "take a message, and I'll call back."

She apologized and recommended a surgeon within the institution to have it "taken care of." At this point, I was told, the cancerous cells had penetrated the derma to a point where it was deemed medically necessary to do radioactive tracing to see if it had metastasized through the lymphatic system—a surgically invasive procedure to remove a lymph node from the axilla (armpit), checking for any cancer cell migration. If this had been addressed at an earlier stage, say six months earlier, it very well could have been treated with a simple excision at the site. Too late, oh that hurt.

I'm hesitant at this point to move forward with this invasive procedure and very untrusting of the medical profession after all the improprieties I have seen over the years from behind the curtain. I get a quick, independent second opinion nonetheless.

The physician assistant (PA) from the private dermatology office where I went for this second opinion tells me that to take another biopsy would disrupt the lymphatic pathways and render useless the radio chemo tracing to see which path the cancer cells would likely follow in the event of malignancy. The rest of the procedure is straightforward standard protocol for the particular depth of cancer cell penetration of the derma shown by the original biopsy. I had made it clear that the reason I was getting a second opinion was because I do not trust the hospital in which I work and who wants to treat. I have seen what they are capable of: it is unsettling. Nevertheless, the PA knows and speaks highly of the oncologist surgeon recommended to me by the nurse practitioner from the dermatology clinic. So I agree to go see her with the sole intent of an information-gathering foray at that point to make as much of an informed decision as possible to how my family and I might go about addressing this new development in our lives.

I hear good things about this surgeon as I'm making my way through the system. I run into employees I've worked with at different points over the years that tell me she, this surgeon, is compassionate and kind. During our meeting the doctor was very pleasant and personable and friendly, using many of her people skills to warm me up and comfort my concerns. She was very good at it. She presented studied published research information as to the risks and benefits of doing and not doing the exploratory procedure. This is around the time the doctor says (aware I'm an employee): "We take care of our own." What does that mean? Did she say that to give me comfort or something else? Do we not treat all patients the same?

I already knew the answer to this: No, not. I know this from firsthand experience. While working I was expected, by management, to give various grades of care depending on who the patient was or who they knew—it is true: I was non-compliant; I treated all my patients equally to the best of my ability with the tools and resources available to me at the time. Integral integrity. As time went on in this institution, the tools, time, and resources diminished as the tasks augmented into very dangerous and inadequate patient care.

What crossed my mind after hearing the doctor say this was: "is this how the system works?" We pay a lot of money for health insurance, and the hospital pays even more on the employees' behalf (I am led to believe, anyway), so is it the institution run as a business looking for opportunities to increase proceeds via procedures? I know, as we have already gone over, that the hospital does a lot of unnecessary testing's and procedures just to raise revenues.

Just the same, I had told the doctor that, if opting for the surgical procedure, even if the node comes back positive, if the cancer had metastasized, I would probably not go any further with treatment. She begins to explain that treatments have come a long way recently, "but we can cross that bridge if and when we come to it."

So now here I am looking at going to nuclear medicine, getting a radioactive dye injected into my circulatory system and getting x-rays shot into my body for a period of time, something like 30 to 40 minutes. Then a few days later they will render me unconscious with drugs, artificially ventilate me (I specifically requested that anesthesia not intubate but use an LMA instead; I had already cleared that with the surgeon. Whether this was reality or not I'll probably never know. "What happens in the OR stays in the OR."), and cut into my lower forearm making two incisions there, one on each side of the cancerous growth about six inches long and taking out a chunk of skin about an inch wide in an almost football-like shape to make for smoother shin reattachment with no "buckles" of skin upon healing. Then to my armpit to cut open a view of the lymph nodes below the surface, find the radioactive nodes, and take one or two out to send to the lab for analysis, looking for metastatic cancer cells.

She did a nice job and, as it turned out, I am one of the luckier ones who, after-the-fact, can question whether it is all just a big scam to raise revenue or heroics. As I like to say, "the facility and the equipment are not cheap. It needs to be paid for, sitting idle does not pay the bills," and I, and the hospital, had paid a lot of insurance premiums over the years. The lymph node came back negative. Yet I will always be left to wonder: what did the doctor mean when she exclaimed, "we take care of our own?"

CONCLUSION

Corporate America has made us deathly ill and the institution of "Healthcare" has swooped in to devour before the kill.

Institutions are failing us by greed of money. Curb the greed and be more equitable with resources. Cap salaries. Antiquity has something to say about this conduct of a social affair.

The Tao: "By not exalting the talented, you will cause the people to cease from rivalry and contention." Practice "non-Ado." No one being exalted, no one glorified. All encouraged and promoted to their individual strengths, preferably all to their unique vocations. All receiving the same compensation for a job well done; dedication to their own specific "God"-given talents in contribution to the community in which we all live; no matter whether large or small. Each has their own "shit" to deal with for the health, wellbeing, and happiness toward a peaceful, tranquil life for all. The farming Founding Fathers of this country understood the advantages of the community all working together to meet common goals for the health and wellbeing of all. They seemed to have learned through antiquity to put all that shit to good use fertilizing new growth. These advanced farmers of their day knew that without the group's wellbeing, as one whole, the "cogs," if you will, will have nothing to hold on to and spin off into oblivion. They knew their history; they studied past attempts at organizations governing peoples, large and small, vast and wide. They knew, after many long, heated debates that they had come up with an imperfect system of governance yet felt it was the best they could agree upon — ratified with much deliberation and consternation. Yet, still, the focus was on the health and wellbeing of the community as a whole.

Help people die with dignity, love and compassion.

All must turn their faces toward God. Of course, this has already been known for a very long time in relation to the human existence. The problem arises as to whose definition of God one adheres. This, too, is "nothing new under the sun: Vanity of Vanities."

"Unless the lord build the house they labor in vain who build" *Psalm 127*

In the shadow of God:

BEZALEL

Made in the USA
Columbia, SC
22 July 2019